PRAISE FOR *PREGNANT, FIT AND FABULOUS*

There a variety of associated health benefits to exercise during pregnancy for both the mother and her unborn child/children. However, my recent studies have shown that many women are actually reducing their exercise during pregnancy, which is why Mary Bacon's book is like a breath of fresh air. She gently shows the mother-to-be in a clear and concise manner, how vital exercise and diet is and importantly, how it impacts her unborn child. I wouldn't hesitate to recommend this easy-to-read guide for any current or future mother.

~ Dr. Mel Hayman, Ph.D. (CQUniversity), Queensland, Australia

My personal experience in working with Mary Bacon is that she is a true expert in the pre and post natal field. Whether you are a world class athlete like me or a regular mum, you will greatly benefit from her expertise. Mary has a great ability to make pregnancy fitness simple and easy to follow. You too will enjoy this book as much as I did.

~ Jana Pittman, Olympic Medalist, dual World Champion and Commonwealth Games Gold Medalist

Mary Bacon is a highly skilled personal trainer with many years' experience. The book is excellently written and well researched and it will be of great help to any expectant mother!

~ Stephen Giulieri B. App. Sci

pregnant fit and FABULOUS

Your Complete Guide to Exercise Before, During and After Pregnancy

Mary Bacon

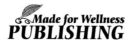

Made for Wellness PUBLISHING

Made For Wellness Publishing
Made For Success Publishing
P.O. Box 1775
Issaquah, WA 98027
www.MadeforSuccessPublishing.com

GOKO Management and Publishing
PO Box 7109
McMahons Point NSW 2060
Australia
www.GOKOPublishing.com

Distributed by Made For Success Publishing in coorperation with GOKO Publishing, Australia.

Library of Congress Cataloging-in-Publication data

Bacon, Mary
   Pregnant, Fit and Fabulous: Your Complete Guide to Exercise Before, During and After Pregnancy

ISBN: 978-1-61339-857-9
LCCN: 2015920984

Book Designed by DeeDee Heathman
Printed in the USA and Australia

*I dedicate this book to my daughters Alexandra and
Stephanie, and my adorable grandson Ryder.*

*You have been there through my greatest and my toughest times. Your
ever consistent love, encouragement and support means the world to me
and is a real blessing. You will always be my greatest achievement.*

CONTENTS

MAJOR MUSCLES OF THE BODY

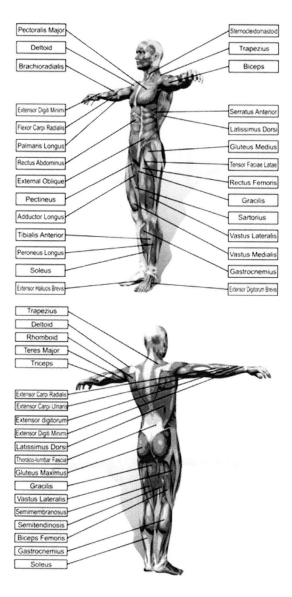

Throughout this book, I will frequently refer to muscles by name. I have placed it here for easy reference.

BIRTHING THIS BOOK

As a personal trainer, my extensive professional qualifications are complemented by an even more important role: the proud mother of my two beautiful daughters, Alexandra, twenty-six and Stephanie, twenty-four. From this standpoint, I feel competent and comfortable in assisting, training and guiding women (and their partners) to happily and confidently adapt to the at times overwhelming physical and emotional experiences that accompany having a baby.

Whether your goal is to fall pregnant, prepare your body for your next pregnancy, or to encourage a family member or friend to do so, this book is for you. Through all the stages of pregnancy, this book will guide you and your partner to a healthier, happier you from before you conceive, during pregnancy and post-pregnancy. You will discover how exercise will make you mentally, emotionally and physically fit. You will have more energy, feel fitter and be healthy and strong.

For a successful and healthy pregnancy and delivery as well as being a positive experience, it is vital that the mother-to-be has positive thoughts and emotions, as these produce beneficial chemicals in the brain. This will naturally have a flow-on effect to your baby. In addition, positive thoughts and emotions will help your partner to support and encourage you. Both parents should have the mental and emotional mantra of "positive mother – happy and healthy baby".

Your child will have attributes, personality, genes, etc. from your partner as well, so making sure he is fit and healthy is almost as important as it is for you – the expectant mother.

As far as the effect of pregnancy on parents is concerned, women may think the weight gained during pregnancy will be lost automatically after their first child, and only after several pregnancies do they realise that the excess weight remains and even accumulates.

Shorter labour, fewer C-sections: The same study also discovered that the exercising women's active labour was two hours shorter and the incidence of operative delivery was reduced from 48 to 14 per cent.

Women who exercised regularly during their pregnancies reported less depression, daily hassles and pregnancy-specific stress in the first and second trimesters.[1] The American College of Obstetrics and Gynaecologists (ACOG) adds that a return to physical activity after pregnancy has been associated with decreased incidence of postpartum depression.[2]

Exercising during pregnancy can not only lead to a quicker recovery but a quicker return to pre-pregnancy weight as well, according to studies by James Clapp of Case Western Reserve University (USA).[3]

The benefits of adopting a positive approach to lifestyle change through nutrition and exercise will last long after your baby is born. I strongly encourage you to explore this book further and stay open to the ideas it offers.

This book has been written especially for you! The time you invest in these pages can literally change your life!

---

1   Journal of Psychosomatic Obstetrics and Gynaecology, 2003

2   ACOG Committee Opinion No.267, Exercise During Pregnancy and the Postpartum Period, January 2002

3   Source Australian Fitness Network e-news IHRSA published 27th July, 2004.

CHAPTER 1

BE READY TO GET PREGNANT!

W e live in a high-tech, fast-paced world these days, and obtaining information on web, e-books, blogs or podcasts has proven a huge advantage. However, as a pregnant mother or post pregnancy, finding the *right* advice and exercises can be a huge challenge. In my personal experience, parents are making decisions that are more educated on these matters, and want to do everything possible to have a healthy baby.

In my 20 years' experience in the Fitness Industry, there has been a radical change in the attitude towards exercise during pregnancy. The days are long gone when women were told to endure the discomforts of pregnancy.

Publications from the American College of Obstetricians and Gynaecologists (ACOG) provide new recommendations and guidelines for exercise and the postpartum period (immediately after the birth). For example, a new finding by the ACOG[4] suggests that exercise can help in the prevention and management of gestational diabetes.

According to the Australian Diabetes Council, losing 5-7% of excess weight and participating in 150 minutes of moderate intensity exercise each week, can reduce the risk of type 2 diabetes by 60%. Gestational diabetes occurs in 5-8% of Australian women (at least 17,000) during pregnancy. Gestational diabetes usually develops around the 24th to 28th week. Although gestational diabetes usually disappears after the baby is born, women who've had gestational diabetes have a 10 times greater risks of developing type 2 diabetes in the future.

Because pregnant women are more open to changing their behaviour for the benefit of their baby, pregnancy presents a unique opportunity to introduce positive behaviour modifications. For example, women may cease smoking or reduce their alcohol intake in order to nurture their

---

4   Source: Australian Fitness Network Magazine, Current guidelines for exercise and pregnancy – Spring 2005

unborn child. Pregnant women are receptive to health advice and will usually listen to and willingly follow their doctor and trainer's recommendations regarding lifestyle and behaviour changes.

Creating an environment of love and getting ready to create life is a very exciting time. After your baby is born, a supportive environment where your partner is available for you emotionally and to assist you with such things as cooking, bottle feeding baby, or to help out with things like shopping and cleaning, is so important.

DO YOU NEED TO LOSE WEIGHT BEFORE YOU TRY TO FALL PREGNANT?

Obesity is increasing rapidly all over the world, affecting more than one billion people worldwide.[5] More and more studies have shown that excess weight has a significant contribution towards infertility, especially for women.

One such study is by Dr Jan Willem van der Steeg, a medical researcher in Obstetrics and Gynaecology at the Academic Medical Centre in Amsterdam, who investigated the effects of obesity on spontaneous pregnancy in 3,029 couples between 2002 and 2004 in 24 hospitals in the Netherlands.[6]

Fertility history, height, weight, smoking habits and other medical history was taken at the start of the study and the couples were followed up until they fell pregnant, or had fertility treatment within 12 months.

This study of the research, which compared conception with body mass index (BMI), revealed that pregnancy success rates decline in direct proportion to a woman's weight. It also showed that obesity also affects the chance of spontaneous pregnancy in women who are ovulating normally.

---

5   Haslam and James, 2005

6   Obesity affects spontaneous pregnancy chances in subfertile, ovulatory women, Human Reproduction (2008) 23 (2): 324-328.

I have a great deal of sympathy and empathy for women who are suffering in silence. This is a very challenging and emotional time for women. From an emotional perspective, being overweight takes a huge toll on self-esteem. The ability to exercise can be limited because it's hard to mentally and physically motivate yourself to get moving – even if it's walking. Inactivity can cause a sore back and tight muscles, which can be demotivating for anyone. Lower social economic regions can also contribute, as sometimes the finances are not there to get help with dieticians, or personal trainers or to even have decent fresh food. You may think you have a big frame and that everyone will be looking at you in judgement. So the choice to stay overweight is easier, we see comfort in food, it's a safe place and we keep the mentality of "one day when I lose a bit of weight" I will exercise.

Do not lose heart; there are many places for you to start.

Doing some basic stretches so that you can start mobilising your body will help you start to feel on top of the world. Your mood will begin to lift and you will want to choose better foods and learn portion control.

When starting an aerobic exercise program, previously sedentary women should begin with 15 minutes of continuous exercise three times a week, increasing gradually to 30-minute sessions 4 times a week.[7]

One great and inexpensive way is to go to water aerobics classes, as the water supports 80% of your body weight.

This is why I have specifically addressed the "absolute beginner" so that you can start doing the basics in the privacy of your own home. This will be a safe environment for you, and you just need to get tough with yourself and start believing that you *can* achieve anything and that you can have a healthy body to deliver a healthy baby.

Because you have picked up this book, I am confident that when you do fall pregnant, you will be more aware of healthy weight gain, exercise will become a habit and you can look forward to feeling fantastic. I know

---

7   Davies, Wolfe, Mottola and MacKinnon in a reprint and modified article from the Canadian Society for Exercise Physiology

with some people, the contrast from feeling overwhelmed with being overweight to feeling fit and fabulous has been simply amazing.

After the birth, again you will focus on getting back into shape, and simultaneously choosing to exercise. Remember, when you exercise your energy will soar, and your emotional condition will greatly improve.

If you choose to breast feed, please do not diet! Your body should have enough in the stores to feed the baby, however taking up exercise will greatly increase your fitness level and also help you get your pre-baby shape back. Do not be fooled by the celebrity crash diets and pictures. Most are nutritionally deficient and unhealthy for you and your baby! Drinking lots of purified water, enjoying fresh foods and exercising is your best choice. I must stress the point of "portion distortion" even with healthy, fresh food - just because it is healthy food does not mean it is fine to go back for seconds or thirds.

LIFESTYLE CHOICES – SMOKING!

Cigarette smoke contains many highly poisonous compounds and nicotine is proven to damage brain cell quality. Nicotine can kill brain cells and stop new ones forming in the hippocampus, a brain region involved in memory, according to a French research team. Their finding might explain the cognitive problems experienced by many heavy smokers during withdrawal, they say.[8]

Some research indicates that the accumulation of carbon monoxide in the foetal blood stream could lead to serious reduction in oxygen to the developing infant. Researchers are now finding that smoking mothers are more likely to have hyperactive (ADHD) children, lower test scores and reduced auditory processing in schoolchildren. It is said that tobacco relieves stress and relaxes and here is why: The massive quantities (42,000 ppm) of carbon monoxide that tobacco smoke contains, result in an impaired oxygen supply to the brain, leading to the feeling of drowsiness. This is "cerebral anoxia." It occurs cell by cell, neuron by

8   Source: http://www.newscientist.com/article/dn2286-nicotine-stops-new-brain-cells-forming.html

neuron, year after year. When "...the oxygen supply is cut off, then damage to neurones occurs after a few minutes. Some neurones die".[9]

Dr Geoff Davies, a UK based GP, states that the results of the study demonstrated a disturbing trend among mothers-to-be.[10] Links have been made between prenatal smoking and stunted development in the womb, including bowel and spinal problems, and an increased possibility of suffering respiratory problems in later life.

The research, by the Cardiff Study of All Wales and North West England Twins (CaStANET)[11], concluded smoking during pregnancy almost certainly increased two conditions developing the child: Antisocial Behaviour and ADHD (Attention Deficit Hyperactivity Disorder).

The report concluded, "Maternal prenatal smoking is associated with both antisocial behaviour and ADHD in offspring.

"We cannot conclude with confidence that smoking during pregnancy is not a direct risk factor for both ADHD symptoms and conduct disorder in offspring

"Therefore, the safest clinical message is that smoking in pregnancy should be avoided."[12]

Cigarette smoking elevates your heart rate significantly during exercise. If you are a smoker, your heart rate is elevated even at rest without any kind of activity or exercise. An embryo at 9 weeks would normally have a heart rate of around 160 beats per minute. If your heart rate is accelerated, imagine your baby's!

---

9   Anthony Hopkins, Epilepsy: The Facts (Oxford and New York: Oxford University Press, 1981, cited in http://medicolegal.tripod.com/preventbraindamage.htm

10 Dr G Davies, 1 August 2005

11 A longitudinal research program of child and adolescent development.

12 http://health.dailynewscentral.com/content/view/0001402/62/

Based on this and other overwhelming evidence, I strongly believe and advise that tobacco smoking should be avoided altogether, especially by a pregnant woman.

LIFESTYLE CHOICES – ALCOHOL!

I am very concerned that some mothers-to-be still have a glass of wine or alcoholic drink on regular basis.

One of the longest running studies into the effects of alcohol on the unborn child was conducted by scientists at Harvard Medical School.

The study looked at nearly 480 mothers who were recruited at their first prenatal clinic visit and examined their children six times to age 19.

They found that pregnant women who had three or more units of alcohol a day had babies with a lower height, weight, weight-for-height/ BMI and head circumference than light or non-drinkers, with the effects lasting well past infancy and into young adulthood.

Of the 85 pregnant women classed as heavy drinkers, 17 gave birth to children with Foetal Alcohol Spectrum Disorder, while a further 22 exhibited partial symptoms.

Lead author Dr Robert Carter said the effects could be permanent and affect brain development, giving children a lower IQ for life.[13]

So girls, keep your weight in a healthy range and make healthy life-style choices that will set you up to maximise your exercise routine so you can have an enjoyable and successful pregnancy. Not only will you and your baby benefit greatly, but the rewards will continue well into the future.

---

13 Carter, R. C., Jacobson, J. L., Sokol, R. J., Avison, M. J. and Jacobson, S. W. (2012), Fetal Alcohol-Related Growth Restriction from Birth through Young Adulthood and Moderating Effects of Maternal Prepregnancy Weight. Alcoholism: Clinical and Experimental Research.

CHAPTER 2

TRAINING BEFORE FALLING PREGNANT FOR BOTH PARTNERS

I encourage both partners to look at one year as a reasonable time to develop a motivated exercise regime. Empower yourself with positive self-talk and keep your goals in mind to motivate you. In relation to maternal weight control, there is evidence to suggest that women who exercise before pregnancy and continue to do so during pregnancy tend to weigh less and gain less weight than controls.[14]

However, a meta-analysis of all the available evidence up to 1990 found no effect of exercise on maternal weight gain.[15] This conclusion probably reflects the difficulties of conducting research in this area, as energy intake and expenditure, which are difficult to control in pregnancy studies, affects weight gain. Controlling weight gain during pregnancy is however an important public health priority, because for many women, pre-pregnancy weight is not recovered and the weight which is gained during pregnancy could therefore signal the onset of "creeping obesity" and its associated health problems.[16] Since Australia is currently facing an epidemic of overweight and obesity, attempts to encourage women to remain active during and following pregnancy should be supported.[17]

---

14 Mittlemark, Dorey and Kirschbaum 1991

15 Lockey et al, 1991

16 Wiliamson, Madans, Pamuk et al 1994

17 (Used with permission from Sports Medicine of Australia (SMA) sma.org.au/wp-content/uploads/2009/05/pregnancystatement.pdf

What are the Benefits to Exercise?

☑ Better self-image.
☑ High energy levels – endorphins (feel good hormone).
☑ Fit and healthy body.
☑ Toned and strong body.
☑ Better sleep.
☑ Better sexual relationship with partner.
☑ Better emotional state (increased serotonin and dopamine levels -avoid depression).
☑ Correct BMI (body mass index – weight to height ratio).
☑ Avoid diabetes.
☑ Avoid high blood pressure.
☑ Avoid breast and colon cancer, and many more.

If a woman has a waist of 35 inches or 89 cm or more, she is at greater risk of heart disease.

Colon cancer is on the rise even in young women. It is very important to have a healthy diet, high in fibre with loads of water, before and during pregnancy.

What are the Risks Associated with Not Exercising During Pregnancy?

The following risks increase without exercise during pregnancy:

☒ Loss of muscle tone and fitness level.
☒ Substantial weight increase sometimes leading to obesity.
☒ Risk of gestational diabetes.
☒ Risk of getting high blood pressure or pregnancy-induced hypertension.
☒ Lower back pain.
☒ Emotional highs and lows; not coping with the physical changes.
☒ May develop varicose veins or deep vein thrombosis.
☒ Relationship challenge – leading to depression.
☒ Low self-esteem – leading to depression.[18]

---

18 Wolfe and Mottola 2000

MY PERSONAL STORY

My own story of exercise and pregnancy is a little unusual. I was married at 18, fell pregnant with my first daughter at 19 (totally unplanned but overjoyed) and I was panicking. I thought, *Oh no – this is how I get fat and ugly!*

The thought frightened the daylights out of me. I was so young; I couldn't even confess my fear to my husband. All I could think of was a big fat stomach, big buttocks, chunky thighs and arms.

So, I thought I had to put a plan into action. I had no clue about fitness, exercise, what food to eat or not, what exercises were safe... nothing! At the time, I worked in the city and was catching the train home. During my train trip, I would secretly read a baby magazine by the *Australian Women's Weekly*[19] (this is in 1988!). It had month-by-month pictures of embryo, foetus and baby, and what I was to expect. I was really fascinated and excited by it all, but I felt anxious. I managed to stick to the weight recommendations and was very careful with my food intake. My mission was to walk home from the train station, which was 8km... thankfully it was in the middle of summer and the days were long. We lived in a very safe area in Sydney, so I felt relaxed and happy that I could walk home every day. I did that for as long as I could. I didn't have any pre or post-natal classes to go to or YouTube videos with which to educate myself.

These days there is so much more information and support available for first time mums and I really encourage you to take advantage of it. My encouragement to you is that even if you just start walking, you will still benefit.

After 9 months, Alexandra was born. I joined a gym in the city and soon became hooked on aerobics classes. Shortly after that, I qualified as an aerobics instructor when – lo and behold – a few months later I was

---

19 The ***Australian Women's Weekly*** is an Australian monthly women's magazine published by Bauer Media Group in Sydney. It was first published as a weekly magazine in 1933 by Frank Packer.

pregnant with my second daughter at 21. Arrrgh! Just when I thought I was getting fit, my body blows out again.

The second time around was not so good for me. I know what it's like to not have the energy, I know what it's like to want to sleep for 2 days, and I know what it's like to crave sweet things to comfort myself.

Weight gain during pregnancy

According to the Royal Hospital for Women in Victoria, Australia, weight gain during pregnancy varies. Average weight increase is between 11.5 and 16kg. The usual pattern of weight gain is 1-2kg during the first 3 months, followed by 0.4kg per week or 1-2kg per month during the final six months of pregnancy.

Post Natal weight gain

An American study of 622 women from the time they enrolled for prenatal care until 1 year after the birth highlights the importance of exercise before, during and after pregnancy in controlling long-term weight gain.

Overweight mothers who exercise daily a year after the birth of their first child are on average, 12 pounds lighter than overweight mothers who rarely work out. Women in the study who restricted their food intake after pregnancy were almost four pounds lighter one year after birth than women who did not. And women who were still breastfeeding a year after birth were almost three pounds lighter than women who were not.

Maintaining a positive "can do" attitude toward regular exercise and controlling food intake – that researchers describe as "self-efficacy" – help take off gestational weight gain, which is critical for women's health.

"A woman's intention during pregnancy to exercise after delivery, as well as her confidence in her ability to exercise frequently, were the strongest predictors as to whether women would exercise frequently and lose weight after giving birth," says Christine Olson, professor of nutritional sciences at Cornell University.

The researchers recommend that practitioners "strengthen exercise self-efficacy by providing postpartum women with mastery experiences of setting realistic exercise goals... and food intake self-efficacy by modelling strategies that women can use to avoid overeating in stressful situations."[20]

When training clients, I use the Body Mass Index (BMI), which is a measurement of your body weight to height ratio. I must stress that **this does not apply to body builders and pregnant women.** Only use this chart pre-pregnancy and after eight weeks post pregnancy. Regardless of breastfeeding or not, the measure of your BMI is a good indicator for setting a goal for your target weight.

20 Hinton and Olson, Postpartum Exercise and Food Intake: The Importance of Behavior-Specific Self-efficacy, Journal of the American Dietetic Association, December 2001

BMI	19	20	21	22	23	24	25	26	27	28	29	30	31	32	33	34	35
Height feet									**Body Weight lbs**								
4'10"	90	97	99	106	110	115	119	123	130	134	139	143	148	152	159	161	168
4'11"	95	99	104	108	115	119	123	128	132	139	143	148	152	159	163	168	172
5'00"	97	101	108	112	119	123	128	132	139	143	148	152	159	163	168	174	179
5'01"	99	106	110	117	121	126	132	137	143	148	152	159	163	170	174	181	185
5'02"	104	108	115	119	126	130	137	141	148	152	159	163	170	174	181	185	192
5'03"	108	112	119	123	130	134	141	146	152	159	163	170	174	181	185	192	196
5'04"	110	117	121	128	134	141	146	150	157	163	170	174	181	185	192	196	205
5'05"	115	119	126	132	139	143	150	157	161	168	174	181	185	192	198	205	209
5'06"	119	123	130	137	141	148	154	161	168	172	179	185	192	198	205	209	216
5'07"	121	126	134	141	146	152	159	165	172	179	185	192	198	205	212	216	223
5'08"	126	130	139	143	150	159	163	172	176	183	190	196	203	209	216	223	229
5'09"	128	134	141	150	154	161	170	176	183	190	196	203	209	216	223	229	236
5'10"	132	139	146	152	161	168	174	181	187	194	203	209	216	223	229	236	243
5'11"	137	143	150	157	165	172	179	185	194	201	207	216	223	229	236	243	249
6'00"	141	148	154	161	170	176	183	192	198	205	214	220	227	236	243	249	258
6'01"	143	150	159	165	174	183	190	196	205	212	218	227	236	243	249	258	265
6'02"	148	154	163	172	179	185	194	203	209	218	225	234	240	249	256	265	271
6'03"	152	161	168	176	183	192	201	207	216	225	231	240	247	256	265	271	280
6'04"	157	163	172	181	190	196	205	214	220	229	238	247	254	262	271	280	287
BMI	19	20	21	22	23	24	25	26	27	28	29	30	31	32	33	34	35
	Normal Weight						**Overweight**					**Obesity**					

☒ If your BMI is less than 20, you need to gain weight, and if it is greater than 25 you need to lose weight (unless you are pregnant).

Now that you have this invaluable information, I want to inspire you and toughen you up to embrace and apply this knowledge for yourself and for your baby. So think positive and resolve yourself that you need to exercise. Make the decision to get fit and see yourself pregnant, fit and fabulous!

---

21 Source: www.whathealth.com Used with permission.

CHAPTER 3

YOUR FITNESS PROGRAM BEFORE PREGNANCY

I t is important that you know right up front that it's **never too late** to start your fitness regime. This chapter outlines how to embark on a fitness program, and is suitable for women before pregnancy and also for their partner.

HOW DO I GET STARTED?

Before embarking on any exercise routine, consult with your medical professional and explain that you are committing to start an exercise program. They will give you some basic guidelines to ensure you begin safely. An injury will only demotivate you and distance you from your goals, so it's well worth the extra effort it takes to begin properly.

Your training can be as simple as walking, swimming or golfing through hiring a personal trainer and really getting healthy and strong for your family. There are so many ways you can make getting fit a fun and enjoyable experience. When you find the right activities for you, you will be able to maintain and enjoy the benefits well into the future, and the quality of your life will improve beyond what you can imagine.

In choosing your exercises, I recommend that you choose functional training wherever possible. This means that you perform exercises that are going to give you the strength for your daily functions. Squats, lunges or pushing a pram or trolley can be our daily activity. How many times do you sit down and get up? How many times do you get in and out of your car? Do you squat or lunge while you're putting your washing on the clothes line? I want to prepare you now and train you before you fall pregnant, so that when you are doing your pregnancy program, it will be awesome to see you maintain your figure and only have the bulge at the front!

In designing the exercise programs in this book, I am using the FITT formula, which stands for Frequency, Intensity, Type and Time of exercise.

The Program Charts at the end of the book will also help you to get started.

All exercise sessions follow the general training principles of **Frequency, Intensity, Time and Type (F.I.T.T.)**

TABLE 2: THE FITT PRINCIPLE

Frequency	3-5 days
Intensity	60-80% of your maximum heart rate (MHR) or (12-17) AND "talk test"
Time	30-90 minutes maximum
Type	Cardiovascular, Resistance, Sport specific training, Yoga, Pilates etc.

Frequency: To gain maximum benefit, you will need to work out 3-5 times per week.

Intensity:

- **Cardiovascular** exercise should be at 60 to 80% of your maximum heart rate. Heart rate (beats per minute) is the primary measure of intensity in cardiovascular training. To determine your maximum heart rate (MHR) you take your age (e.g. 30 years old) away from 220 (220-30=190bpm). To determine your 60% heart rate, multiply 190 x 60%=114 beats per minute. To determine your 80%, multiply 190 x 80% = 152 beats per minute.
- **Resistance** training should be heavy enough to challenge your muscles while maintaining good form to avoid injury.

Time: How long do I need to exercise?

Going by the FITT principle, a minimum of 30 minutes is recommended. This is a very general goal for basic fitness; however I like to see people fit in a good hour into their training sessions 5 times a week.

Consider: with a warm up of 5 minutes, cool down 5 minutes or longer, stretching and the actual workout – it will definitely take up an hour for a good training session. Most aerobics classes last 1 hour. Most weights or resistance training sessions are for 45 minutes. If you choose to do a Yoga or Pilates class once a week – that is usually an hour.

You should aim for a minimum training session of 50 minutes to a maximum of 1hr 45 minutes containing cardiovascular, resistance training and flexibility.

Type: What type of exercise?

In order to build your strength and fitness level, it is best to vary your training. A combination of cardiovascular and resistance training is recommended – remember to check with your doctor first. I am also a big fan of stretching and doing some mobilisation and stability work. So pay attention to my chapters on these, as it will help you gain understanding of how to have a strong, supple and toned body that is pain free.

Cardiovascular, flexibility and resistance training each have their place and are of equal importance. In my programs, there are many choices for you, so choose a program that is appropriate to you for your current goals.

CARDIOVASCULAR EXERCISE

Aerobic (or cardiovascular) exercise is where the body uses oxygen and therefore involves the continued activation of muscle. Aerobic exercise also utilises fat as its energy source. Simple exercises such as power walking, jogging, swimming, rowing, cycling are all-aerobic based and duration should be from 20 minutes to 1 hour.

Aerobic exercise can include activities that use large muscle groups (e.g. legs, chest, and back) in a continuous manner such as walking, stationary cycling and low-impact gym classes. These sessions should be between 20 to 60 minutes in duration.

As mentioned earlier we can measure intensity of cardiovascular exercise by our heart rate, which is measured easily with a heart rate monitor. The other popular method is the "talk test", in which you estimate how easy it is to hold a conversation using the descriptions in the Borg scale.[22]

TABLE 3: BORG RATING OF PERCEIVED EXERTION (RPE)

Rating of Perceived Exertion (RPE)	Description	Intensity Level
7	Easy	
8		
9	Very Light	
10		50% MHR
11	Fairly Light	
12		60% MHR
13	Somewhat Hard	
14		70% MHR
15		
16	Hard	80% MHR
17		
18	Very Hard	90% MHR
19	Very, Very Hard	
20	Exhaustion	

- If you are a beginner, during exercise your exertion rate (RPE) should be at 11. This means that your intensity is fairly light – you can still talk, but it maybe a little uncomfortable.
- Regular exercisers or intermediate population should have an exertion rate between 13 and 16.
- For those who are hard core or advanced, your exertion rate should be between 13 and 17-18.

INTERVAL TRAINING

To increase your fitness, I recommend interval training. Rather than maintaining the same exertion rate for the whole time, you increase the exertion for a short time and then drop back to recover. Repeat this cycle for the session. E.g. run for 30 seconds, and walk for 30 seconds; cycle fast for 1 minute, slow for 30 seconds. Lots of gym bikes come with interval (or Kilimanjaro) programs. Rowing is the same: row hard for 2 minutes, rest for 90 seconds and repeat this for 6 times. Interval training

22 Davies et al 2003

will certainly get your heart rate up, and cycle your exertion rate between 13 and 17-18.

So get fit and enjoy your intensity now – before you fall pregnant!

RESISTANCE TRAINING

Resistance or strength training can include weight training such as squats, lunges, push-ups and lat pull-downs. Sessions should be between 30-45 minutes in duration.

Whether you are an athlete or a first-time mum who is exploring the idea of training for pregnancy, strength training offers multiple benefits. For example, muscle tone improves and metabolic rate increases, which also leads to fat burning after pregnancy. In contrast, aerobic training will benefit your fitness level but doesn't give you the physical and psychological benefits that having improved muscle tone and strength does.

Girls, don't be concerned that you will grow big muscles and look masculine. Our hormonal make up is such that we stay feminine with lean and toned muscles.

Did you know that women have relative strength, in other words we can carry or hold our baby for extended periods of time? However men have maximal strength, meaning they can only lift maximum amounts of weight once or twice. So girls, you are stronger than you think and just because you may not be able to lift the same weight as your partner, appreciate your strength.

STRETCHING

This has to be one of the most neglected, misused and laboured aspects of exercise.

Stretching has many benefits, including increased energy and increased circulation. It also helps your joints stay pain free, improves posture and helps you to de-stress. It encourages better sleep and helps prevent other neck, shoulder, upper and lower back problems.

In short, stretching will help bring your body from feeling tight and stiff to a better daily function and will also help you enjoy your exercises more.

It seems that not many people are concerned about the benefits of stretching and assume it's all a myth. But it's not a myth! Let me show you why your muscles need stretching...

We live in a fast-paced world and often in a stressful environment. Our body gets accustomed to this pace as we push our mental and physical capacity to the limits. Our bodies are a bit like a high performance car that needs tune ups. Tension is felt in our neck muscles, upper and lower back, so it's imperative that you do some stretches to relieve stress and tightness.

Your body was designed is such a way that it's supposed to have strength in some muscles and length in others. For example your quads or thigh muscles need strength to help you sit down or to help you lunge down to pick up your baby or shopping.

Your hamstrings, on the other hand, generally need some serious stretching. These days, our posture tends to be conformed to sitting at a desk. Hence the hamstrings become very tight, on both men and women. So stretching your hamstrings will not only help you release them, but also help your lower back.

Your glutes are another 3 muscles that need strengthening. Having strong glutes will help you alleviate some serious lower back pain. According to some physiotherapists, 80% of back problems are due to weak gluteal muscles.

But you need more than just stretching to have your muscles working effectively and safely.

BENEFITS OF BALANCED MUSCLES

A common problem that I see in people is muscle imbalances. These are caused by muscles being too tight or too weak, and may be corrected by stretching and strengthening the relevant muscles.

Use the following table (4) to identify any postural imbalances. I recommend that you address these as soon as possible and certainly before the end of the first trimester (T1).

If you have a personal fitness trainer, work with him or her to help you correct these imbalances. If you do not have the luxury of a personal trainer, *Table 4* outlines what you should look for and which muscles to take care of before commencing an exercise program.

Some of the muscle terminology may be unfamiliar to you (see Glossary), or you may prefer to visit your physiotherapist or osteopath for correct screening and treatment.

TABLE 4: POSTURAL DISTORTION PATTERN

	Postural distortion	Short/tight muscles	Long/weak muscles
Foot/ankle	Feet externally rotated Pronated at ankle	Soleus/gastrocnemius Soleus/gastrocnemius peroneals	Anterior/posterior tibialis Anterior/posterior tibialis
Knees	Adducted/internally rotated	Adductors – IT band	Gluteus medius Gluteus maximus Hip External Rotators
Hips	Anterior pelvic tilt	Iliopsoas Rectus Femoris Piriformis Erector spinae Latissimus dorsi	Gluteus maximus Gluteus minimus Inner Unit: Transverse Abs Pelvic Floor
Shoulders	Protracted shoulder girdle	Pectoralis major/minor Latissimus dorsi	Scapular retractors: Rhomboids Mid/lower trapezius
Head	Cervic extensors	Sternocleidomastoid Upper trapezius Scalenes Levator scapulae	Deep cervical flexors

In my programs, you will see how to release muscle spasms, stretch tight muscles, and follow with strengthening exercises for weak muscles. You will effectively be following a comprehensive training program that focuses on the strength, stability and corrective techniques to overcome imbalances.

If there is discomfort or pain in any area, you may need the assistance of your osteopath for adjustment.

It is important to understand that if you have already been training for a considerable time with an existing imbalance, then it will take some 3000 repetitions to reverse a faulty movement pattern. Your brain is efficient at programming your movements through training so to correct any issues requires focus and time. Alternatively, not addressing existing imbalances can potentially lead to further problems over time.

Benefits of Stability and Mobility Training

Training your body for stability can be just as important as flexibility or resistance training. In my many years as a trainer I have assessed the functionality and movement of my clients and have found the results have revealed that many people suffer with an unstable pelvis.

Stability training has been overlooked or at the very least, given insufficient attention when writing up programs for individuals at local gyms.

Our focus or obsession with getting fit has bypassed the importance of creating stability in our body, especially in the pelvis area.

You've heard the saying "an ounce of prevention is worth a pound of cure". It's far better to address any potential or existing issues e.g. unstable pelvis, or tight lower back now, rather than developing these issues later in your pregnancy.

Stability training before falling pregnant and focusing on getting the pelvis stable, strong, ready for pregnancy and labour is essential. This is not only in order to correct existing imbalances, but also to prevent further aggravation during and post pregnancy. Only specialised physiotherapists will educate their clients concerning this specific area. Your doctor may not have the time to share this vital information with you, as visits during your pregnancy are focused on your unborn baby's progress, and on making sure other vital statistics are monitored.

- **Internal muscles** like the pelvic floor and multifidus, (deep spine muscle that runs from the base of the skull all the way down to your tailbone) work together to create stability in the pelvis – these are termed **Core** muscles.

- **External muscles** like the gluteus (buttocks) and obliques (waist) must also be strengthened in order to create stability in the body.

Mobility means that your joints and muscles have a good range of movement (ROM) and are not restricted by tightness or stiffness e.g. hips area – tight hip flexors, which may lead to lower back issues.

BUT WAIT THERE'S MORE!

The FITT formula alone won't be enough for you so I am adding another component to your training to improve your results:

RELEASING MUSCLE SPASMS (MYOFASCIAL TRIGGER POINTS)

Before the stretching and strengthening program, we need to address tight spots in certain muscles. I refer to this as "releasing muscle spasms" or "trigger point release", but technically it is known as "myofascial release".

In Latin "*myo*" means muscle, and "*fascia*" means connective tissue.

Myofascial tissue is the loose but strong layer of connective tissue often containing fat that connects from head to toe and covers every muscle in the body. A fascia "band" is a layer of fibrous or connective tissue that surrounds muscles, groups of muscles, blood vessels and nerves. Similar to ligaments and tendons, fascia is dense, regular, connective tissue, containing closely-packed bundles of collagen fibres, orientated in a wavy pattern and parallel to the direction of pull.

Ligaments join bone to bone; tendons join muscle to bone and fascia.

Some research suggests that fascia might be able to contract independently and thus actively influence muscle dynamics. For this reason, it is vital that you look after your fascia as much as your muscle, as fascia does affect muscle movement and your body's performance.

A recent study by The School of Human Kinetics and Recreation at Memorial University of Newfoundland showed self-myofascial release with a foam roller on quadriceps for 2 minutes led to an 8-10% improvement in the range of motion.[23] A few minutes can make a big difference to your stretches and ability to perform exercises properly, so it is well worth taking the time.

Muscles can go into spasm for various reasons; they may be weak, overused or due to bad posture. I highly recommend myofascial releases, which aims to release muscle spasms. A lot of the time we feel we are not flexible and will attempt to do some quick stretches, but this does not give us the desired results. The reason is that a muscle may become dysfunctional as it goes into spasm. This will cause great discomfort and, if left untreated it may become inflamed.

Clinical treatment of localised and radiating muscle pain or *myofascial dysfunction* involves the hands-on treatment of releasing trigger points and often involves the use of direct pressure massage, heat, ice and specific exercises.

To help release these muscle spasms, I will be showing you a simple technique using a foam roller. There will be specific releases for before and after pregnancy (see Group A *Self-Myofascial Release (Muscle Spasm Release) Before and After Pregnancy*) and for during pregnancy (see Group E *Self-Myofascial Release During Pregnancy*). Total time for these will be no more than 10 minutes for the whole body. Be sure to follow the instructions correctly. If the spasms still persist, please see your physiotherapist or health care practitioner for further treatment. Men should do this as well, if they want to achieve a strong and flexible body.

---

23 Macdonald G, Penney M, Mullaley M, Cuconato A, Drake C, Behm DG, Button DC, An Acute Bout of Self Myofascial Release Increases Range of Motion Without a Subsequent Decrease in Muscle Activation or Force., School of Human Kinetics and Recreation, Memorial University of Newfoundland,

CHAPTER 4

WHO CAN AND CANNOT EXERCISE?

Caution!

Before starting any program, ensure that you have medical clearance from your medical support team or obstetrician. I highly recommend that you visit a good osteopath or physiotherapist in order to assess imbalances that may be pre-existing and need correcting.

ACOG recommends that all pregnant women should be encouraged to participate in both aerobic and strength training after medical clearance.[24] Current guidelines recommend 30 minutes of exercise on most, if not all days of the week for women with uncomplicated pregnancies. The women should be well hydrated and perceive the exercise to be mild to moderate.

The following guidelines have been approved by Society of Obstetricians and Gynaecologists (SOGC) Clinical Practice Obstetric Committee and approved by the Executive and Council of the SOGC of Canada, and approved by the Board of Directors of the Canadian Society for Exercise Physiology.

1. All women without contraindications should be encouraged to participate in aerobic and strength-conditioning exercises as part of a healthy lifestyle during their pregnancy.
2. Reasonable goals of aerobic conditioning in pregnancy should be to maintain a good fitness level throughout pregnancy without trying to reach peak fitness or train for an athletic competition.
3. Choose activities that will minimise the risk of loss of balance and foetal trauma.
4. Adverse pregnancy or neonatal outcomes are not increased for exercising women.

---

24 ACOG Committee Opinion No.267, Exercise During Pregnancy and the Postpartum Period, January 2002

5. Initiation of pelvic floor exercises in the immediate postpartum period may reduce the risk of future urinary incontinence.
6. Moderate exercise during lactation does not affect the quantity or composition of breast milk or impact infant growth.

Table 5: Contraindications to exercise during pregnancy, lists contraindications that your doctor will consider before giving medical clearance to exercise. If you become aware that you have any of these conditions, be sure to raise them specifically with your obstetrician before embarking on an exercise regime.

It is a widely accepted fact that fit women have shorter labours with a significantly lower rate of caesarean sections (C-sections). More evidence is showing that women who begin regular, moderate exercise in trimester 1 (T1), and continue throughout their pregnancy will also benefit. One study demonstrated that the first-time mothers who did not exercise were 4.5 times more likely to require a C-section.[25]

WHEN NOT TO EXERCISE

Stop exercising immediately and consult your physician if you experience any of the following symptoms during exercise:

- ☒ Vaginal Bleeding
- ☒ Shortness of breath prior to exertion
- ☒ Dizziness
- ☒ Headache
- ☒ Chest pain
- ☒ Muscle weakness
- ☒ Calf pain or swelling
- ☒ Pre-term labour
- ☒ Decreased foetal movement
- ☒ Amniotic fluid leakage[26]

---

25 Ref: Australian Fitness Network magazine e-news published 27th July, 2004

26 ACOG Committee Opinion No.267, Exercise During Pregnancy and the Postpartum Period, January 2002

You must **NOT** exercise if you suffer with any of the symptoms above or in the tables below. Furthermore, I strongly advise you to refer to your doctor or medical support if you are experiencing any of the symptoms unless you have been cleared by your obstetrician.

TABLE 5: CONTRAINDICATIONS TO EXERCISE DURING PREGNANCY[27]

Absolute Contraindications	Relative Contraindications
☒ Haemodynamically significant heart disease	☒ Severe anaemia
☒ Pregnancy induced hypertension	☒ Unevaluated maternal cardiac arrhythmia
☒ Restrictive lung disease	☒ Mild/moderate cardiovascular disorder
☒ Incompetent cervix/cerclage	☒ Chronic bronchitis
☒ Multiple gestation at risk for premature labour (>= twins)	☒ Heavy smoker
☒ Persistent praevia after 26 weeks gestation	☒ Mild/moderate respiratory disorder
☒ Premature labour during current pregnancy	☒ History of extremely sedentary lifestyle
☒ Ruptured membranes	☒ Extreme morbid obesity
☒ Growth restricted foetus	☒ Extreme underweight
☒ Persistent 2nd and 3rd trimester bleeding	☒ Malnutrition or eating disorder
☒ Uncontrolled type 1 diabetes	☒ Intra-uterine growth restriction/retardation in current pregnancy
☒ Uncontrolled thyroid disease	☒ Previous spontaneous abortion
☒ Other serious cardiovascular or systemic disorder	☒ Previous preterm birth
	☒ Twin pregnancy after 28 weeks
	☒ Poorly controlled type 1 diabetes
	☒ Poorly controlled hypertension/pre-eclampsia
	☒ Poorly controlled seizure disorder
	☒ Poorly controlled thyroid disease
	☒ Orthopaedic limitations
	☒ Other significant medical conditions.

27 Adapted from and used with permission: Liz Dene, Australian Fitness Network Magazine, Spring 2005 / Source: ACOG Committee Opinion No.267, Exercise During Pregnancy and the Postpartum Period, January2002 and Davies, Wolfe, Mottola and MacKinnon in a reprint and modified article from the Canadian Society for Exercise Physiology.

Some of these indications are self-explanatory however the following is a quick outline and description in layman's terms:

Haemodynamically significant heart disease

Routine antenatal screening for congenital malformation is performed as part of the general scan for irregularities at 18-20 weeks gestation. To date, this identifies about 25% of affected foetuses on average. Congenital heart disease is a major cause of death in infancy in term babies.

Incompetent cervix/cerclage

Incompetent cervix is one that opens without labour too early in pregnancy.

Persistent praevia after 26 weeks

Placenta praevia is a low-lying placenta and is one of the leading causes of third-trimester bleeding. It is not common although it may be a dangerous and occasionally fatal condition.

Pregnancy induced hypertension and Poorly controlled hypertension/pre-eclampsia

Pregnancy-induced hypertension (PIH) is a form of high blood pressure in pregnancy occurring in about 5% to 8% of all pregnancies. Pregnancy-induced hypertension is also called toxemia or preeclampsia. Preeclampsia occurs typically after 20 weeks gestation. Appropriate pre-natal care is vital to diagnose and manage blood pressure.

Intra-uterine growth restriction/retardation

IUGR is when a baby is not growing inside the uterus at the normal rate. These babies usually have a low birth weight.

Severe Anaemia

When the number of red blood cells or the amount of haemoglobin (the oxygen-carrying protein) in the blood is lower than expected, it is called anaemia. Women with severe anaemia are more likely to deliver early and have small babies.

Heavy smoker

In addition to the nicotine damage to your developing baby discussed earlier, heavy smoking is a relative contraindication to exercise during pregnancy, which means you may not be allowed to exercise at all.

If you're still smoking when you fall pregnant, please see your doctor for clearance before you start exercise. You can probably guess that your doctor will tell you to give up entirely, so your pregnancy may be just the incentive you need to kick the habit!

Poorly controlled thyroid disease

Thyroid disease is a disorder that affects the thyroid gland. Sometimes the body produces too much or too little thyroid hormone. Thyroid hormones regulate metabolism—the way the body uses energy—and affect nearly every organ in the body. Too much thyroid hormone is called hyperthyroidism and can cause many of the body's functions to speed up. Too little thyroid hormone is called hypothyroidism and can cause many of the body's functions to slow down.

Thyroid hormone plays a critical role during pregnancy both in the development of a healthy baby and in maintaining the health of the mother.

Women with thyroid problems can have a healthy pregnancy and protect their baby's health by learning about pregnancy's effect on the thyroid, keeping current on their thyroid function testing, and taking the required medications.[28]

Cardiac Arrhythmia

Cardiac Arrhythmia is an irregular heartbeat.

---

28 http://www.endocrine.niddk.nih.gov/pubs/pregnancy/

CHAPTER 5

ANATOMICAL AND PHYSIOLOGICAL CHANGES DURING PREGNANCY

M any anatomical and physiological changes during pregnancy have the potential to affect the musculoskeletal system at rest and during exercise.

WEIGHT GAIN

Increased weight in pregnancy may significantly increase the forces across joints such as hips and knees by as much as 100% during weight-bearing exercises like running and squatting. Such large forces may cause discomfort to normal joints and increase damage to previously unstable joints.

POSTURAL DISTORTION PATTERNS

Weight gain plus increased ligamentous laxity due to the rise in oestrogen and relaxin during pregnancy will lead to significant likelihood of "postural distortion patterns", which we discussed in Chapter 3 "Your Fitness Program Before Pregnancy".

Pregnant women typically develop lower back arch (lumbar lordosis), which contributes to the high prevalence (50%) of low back pain. The pelvis often rotates forward (anteriorly) due to the position and weight of the baby. To compensate for the increased lower back arch (lordotic arch), the upper back curves to give a hunched over look (kyphotic curve).

Consequently, the neck (cervical spine) may then be affected, as the shoulders become more rounded and the head will shift forward. Your head weighs 8% of your total body weight. When your head is poking forward (protruding) - for example sitting at a computer - you are doubling the percentage of load through your upper back and down to your lower back.

Men with large stomachs have exactly the same posture and muscular stiffness as a pregnant woman. Left unaddressed, this will cause long term chronic back problems.

Postural distortion patterns should be addressed in T1 to help strengthen you for the trimesters to follow. For help with postural corrections, I recommend both partners follow the recommendations in Chapter 3 "Your Fitness Program Before Pregnancy".

OTHER PHYSIOLOGICAL STATES OF THE PREGNANT WOMAN

BLOOD VOLUME

Blood volume is the total amount of blood within in the body. From 6-8 weeks, blood volume gradually increases up to around 40%, which increases the amount of blood the heart has to pump with each beat. Respiratory rate increases due to greater oxygen demands and consumption. Additional pressure of the uterus on the diaphragm also increases respiratory rate and the general work of breathing. Additional weight adds load to the joints and increases joint stress.

PLASMA VOLUME

Plasma volume is the measure of plasma volume in the blood. It constitutes 55% of blood fluid, is mostly water (92% by volume), and contains proteins, glucose, mineral ions, hormones, carbon dioxide (plasma being the main medium for excretory product transportation), and blood cells themselves. Plasma volume increases gradually over pregnancy, up to around 50% (due to increased sodium and water retention).

CARDIAC OUTPUT

Cardiac output is the volume of blood pumped by the heart per minute. Cardiac output increases by 30-50% by the middle of the third trimester (T3), initially due to increased heart rate, and afterward by an increased stroke volume (controlled to by increased plasma and blood volume).

STROKE VOLUME

Stroke volume is the volume of blood the heart pumps with each beat. Stroke volume increases by 10% by the end of the first trimester (T1) and later up to 35%.

HEART RATE

Heart rate is the number of cardiac contractions by the heart each minute (beats per minute). There is an increase of 10-15 beats/min in resting heart-rate in pregnancy. At rest, heart rate increases by 20% during second and third trimesters (T1 and T2).

BLOOD PRESSURE

Blood pressure is the pressure of the blood in the arteries as it is pumped around the body by the heart. This is the highest reading (e.g. 120 mmHg if your blood pressure is 120/80) and is known as the systolic measurement, which fluctuates with stress, emotion, anxiety and exercise, possibly increasing this reading.

The lower reading is the pressure on the blood vessels between the heart pumps or when the heart is at rest (e.g. 80mmHg if your blood pressure is 120/80), known as the diastolic measurement. The diastolic pressure is the constant, lower pressure on the blood vessels and generally the measurement your doctor focuses on during pregnancy

The smaller arteries in the body can control blood pressure through tightening and relaxing. If they tighten to increase blood pressure, they do not allow blood to flow as freely but this can also reduce oxygen and nutrient flow to the placenta and baby. This is one physical side effect of very high blood pressure during pregnancy called *preeclampsia*.[29]

High blood pressure during pregnancy can be potentially dangerous:

- ☒ **Decreased blood flow to the placenta.** This reduces the baby's supply of oxygen and nutrients, potentially slowing the baby's growth and increasing the risk of a low birth weight.
- ☒ **Placental abruption.** With this condition, the placenta prematurely separates from the uterus. Placental abruption can deprive the baby of oxygen and cause heavy bleeding in the mother.
- ☒ **Premature delivery.** Sometimes an early delivery is needed to prevent potentially life-threatening complications.
- ☒ **Future cardiovascular disease.** Women who develop pre-eclampsia — a serious condition characterised by high blood pressure and protein in the urine after 20 weeks of pregnancy — might be at increased risk of cardiovascular disease later in life, despite the fact that their blood pressure returns to normal after delivery.[30]

RESPIRATORY RATE

Respiratory rate increases 15% (by 2-3 breaths per minute)

OXYGEN CONSUMPTION

Oxygen consumption (VO2) increases by at least 20% (or 50ml/min)

BREATHING CAPACITY

Increased work in breathing – Later in pregnancy breathing requires increased work due to the elevated diaphragm (however, total lung

29 http://www.birth.com.au

30 http://www.mayoclinic.com/health/pregnancy/PR00125

capacity may decrease only slightly due to compensatory increases in transverse and antero-posterior diameters of the chest and flaring of the ribs).[31]

There is an increased blood flow to the lining of the nose and respiratory tract, leading to symptoms of nasal congestion.

NUTRITIONAL CHANGES

Rates of delivery of oxygen and nutrient to the placenta are major regulators of foetal growth. There adequate calorific intake is required.[32]

Pregnant women use carbohydrates at a greater rate, both at rest and during exercise, than non-pregnant women do. After the 13th week of pregnancy, an extra 300 calories per day are required to meet the metabolic needs of pregnancy.[33]

This energy intake is increased:

- When daily energy expenditure increases due to exercise.
- In weight-bearing exercise, the energy requirement progressively increases along with the increase in weight during the course of the pregnancy.

---

31 Ciliberto and Marx 1998

32 Clapp 2006

33 Artal et al 2003

CHAPTER 6

YOUR FITNESS PROGRAM DURING PREGNANCY

The benefits are enormous!

- You will have better delivery of oxygen and nutrients, particularly to your uterus and placenta. (Circulation is another major issue with pregnant women. 'Toxemia of pregnancy' is high blood pressure, which affects 7% of pregnant women.)
- Aerobic exercise improves peristalsis/digestion, which means you are less likely to suffer from constipation and haemorrhoids as well as varicose veins and kidney function problems.
- Weight bearing exercise such as walking/jogging and aerobic weight training will increase bone density.
- Women who exercise during pregnancy experience more weight loss after pregnancy as well as improved overall conditioning.
- Aerobic weight training is not only great for increasing fitness, bone density and toning your body, it will prepare you to tolerate physical stress such as lifting and carrying your baby.

As discussed in Chapter 3 "Your Fitness Program Before Pregnancy", exercise sessions follow the general training principles of **Frequency, Intensity, Time and Type (F.I.T.T.)**. However, the guidelines are modified to suit the different stages of pregnancy.

Take careful note of the modifications below and follow the programs that I have outlined in the "During Pregnancy" chapters.

TABLE 6: THE FITT PRINCIPLE DURING PREGNANCY

Frequency	Most Days
Intensity-using Borg Scale	T1: 12 for the unconditioned pregnant woman T1 and T2: (12-14) T3: (12-14) "talk test"
Time	15 minutes for the unconditioned pregnant woman 30 minutes at correct intensity for trimester
Type	Combination of cardiovascular and resistance training

Frequency and Time of exercise

The two major concerns of exercise during pregnancy is the effect on *thermoregulation* (the maintenance of a steady body temperature despite changes in the environment) and maintaining your *energy balance* (i.e. energy level and quality of your food intake). It is best to limit the duration to 30 minutes maximum, depending on intensity. Another option is to accumulate activity to shorter periods such as 15-minute sessions.

Using the Borg scale described in Chapter 3 "Your Fitness Program Before Pregnancy", the intensity of cardiovascular exercise during pregnancy is much lower. You will also see (RPE) which stands for perceived exertion rate – which is directly related to the Borg Scale.

- Intensity for an unconditioned pregnant woman would be exertion rate of 12. This is a very light intensity and should only be done for 15 minutes.
- Intensity generally for trimesters 1 (T1), trimester 2 (T2) and trimester 3 (T3) should be within the range of 12-14. This is a comfortable pace; however 30 minute workout should feel that you have done a good workout.
- Trimester 3 (T3) for the unconditioned woman – intensity may vary, depending on how comfortable she is.

Having said this, the general low intensity aerobics class or yoga class will run for 60 minutes. Keep in mind that the recommended 30 minutes is only a recommendation that is safe and effective during pregnancy. Please note that the 30-minute time limit ONLY includes cardio and/or weight training. Any stretching or myofascial work is in addition to this time.

Intensity – What Heart Rate during pregnancy?

TABLE 7: MODIFIED HEART RATE TARGET ZONE
FOR AEROBIC EXERCISE IN PREGNANCY[34]

Maternal age	Heart rate target zone (bpm)
<20	140-155
20-29	135-150
30-39	130-145
40+	125-140

Please note: This is an approximation only and will be subject to the fitness level, body weight and which trimester the individual falls into.

Modified heart rate zone has been established, so that women can have this as a guide and check their age and target heart rate during pregnancy. A heart rate monitor is a great tool to invest in.

In the first trimester (T1) there is an increase in maternal heart rate at any given workload, but the rate of perceived exertion (RPE) will be decreased due to an under filling of the cardiovascular system. This means that you may feel like you can increase the intensity of your exercise – however you should NOT do this. The intensity of your workouts should remain low to protect your body from overheating, as weeks 3 to 8 hold the greatest risk of foetal malformation to due heat shock on cell development. From week 8 to 13, all the organs of the baby are developed - so fellas, if your wife or partner is looking tense or not her joyful self, it's due to the fact that she is making liver, kidneys and the rest, and is at her peak of producing baby's organs. Be especially kind to her at this time.

Keep well within the target zone for this period – see *Table 7: Modified heart rate target zone for aerobic exercise in pregnancy* above, so stay sensible.

In the second trimester (T2) you should really enjoy your pregnancy and training. It's the best time to remain consistent with your exercise

---

34 Source: Canadian Society for Exercise.

routine. Morning sickness would have subsided or disappeared altogether by now, and you will feel more like yourself. Your tummy bulge is progressing nicely, and you are able to do most exercises without too much discomfort. Your heart rate should be at the recommended level, and if you are a regular exerciser, your intensity can increase a little during this time (a heart rate monitor is always advisable). Keep within the Borg scale, and don't overdo it.

Past 16 weeks, make sure not to lie on your back for prolonged periods of time, as the blood flow is restricted through the inferior vena cava – which is the large vein that carries blood from the lower half of the body, back up to the right hand side of the heart. When you are doing abdominal exercises on the floor, make sure you turn on your left side for recovery of one minute and then return to the exercise. Also, if you mix your training with 2 aerobics classes per week at a moderate intensity, this works very well. This is especially beneficial as there are a lot of lateral movements (side to side) – which help to work the hips muscles, while keeping the pelvis stable.

In the third trimester (T3) there is a decrease in maternal heart rate at any given workload; however, the perceived exertion rate (RPE) increases because the heart circulates a higher volume of blood and the increased maternal weight. Most women find it difficult to keep up the exercise intensity as their pregnancy progresses due to the growth of the baby. Many mums are exhausted even thinking about exercise at this stage, let alone doing any exercise.

Research done by Associate Professor Dr Lene A H Haakstad, PhD, at the Norwegian School of Sport Sciences found that most common reasons for performing regular exercise in the third trimester (T3) were a positive impact on health complaints and increase in physical fitness. A number of women also believed that performing regular exercise would improve their well-being, contribute to the reduction of pregnancy complaints, and help prevent excessive weight gain.

The most frequently reported barriers towards exercise were: pregnancy complaints; lack of time; too much effort to get started and childcare difficulties.

It is important to form good exercise habits before pregnancy. Of 262 women reporting to be non-exercisers pre-pregnancy, only 9 started a regular exercise program and were defined as regular exercisers in the third trimester (T3). Women who decreased regular exercise in the third trimester (T3) had a higher weight gain and reported having no good social role model with regard to exercise behaviour during childhood. Pre-pregnancy physical inactivity was the strongest predictor of decreased maternal exercise in the third trimester (T3).

According to research conducted in Canada, women who develop diabetes during pregnancy can reduce their need for insulin treatment by participating in resistance training program.

Approximately 1 out of every 2 pregnant women will experience lower back pain during their pregnancy, more commonly after the 6-month stage. As the baby grows, the mother's centre of gravity shifts forward, increasing the curvature of the lower back (*lumbar lordosis*). As the abdominal muscles stretch, muscle tone diminishes and the mother will find maintaining a neutral posture increasingly difficult. This is why strength training for the deep abdominal wall together with back strengthening and stretching exercises is highly beneficial.

Pregnant women should be able to continue their strength training routine throughout pregnancy. It is important to remember to breathe normally when working out because holding your breath can reduce oxygen delivery to the placenta. To keep the oxygen supply going, avoid maximum lifts and heavy resistances, especially when the hormone relaxin is present in increased amounts. Relaxin production occurs naturally in the pregnant mother and provides increased movement in the pelvis to accommodate the growing baby and allow for an easier birth. Relaxin concentration is greatest in the first trimester, drops after 4 months and peaks again during labour.

Type of exercise

Cardiovascular

During pregnancy, I recommend you mix cardiovascular and weight (strength) training.

Choose low impact forms of aerobic exercise such as walking, low impact aerobic classes, water aerobics. Swimming is an excellent form of aerobic exercise during pregnancy. The water supports 80% of your body weight, allowing you to feel comfortable and still have an efficient work out. This is a total body workout and fantastic for the deep abdominal wall.

Strength training

You should continue your strength training during pregnancy, but the focus changes to be more about being strong and fit to carry your growing baby and for the delivery. Many of the exercises are similar, but be sure to follow the modifications carefully. I have outlined which exercises are suitable for each trimester in *Table 16: Strengthening Exercises During Pregnancy*.

Postural

- When lying on your back (supine position) during pregnancy, cardiac output (the volume of blood pumped by the heart) is decreased because of the increased pressure on the inferior vena cava (large vein). This causes a decrease in blood flow back to your heart.
- In the standing position, the pelvic vessels are increasingly compressed as the baby grows, which also impairs venous (blood) return. Minimise a prolonged standing position, as it prevents the calf muscles from assisting with venous (blood) return.
- Be aware of posture, end range of movement (beyond normal limits) and joint stability. Instability in the pelvis and tightness of the surrounding musculature can lead to such issues as sacroiliac joint pain (tailbone) and pubic symphysis instability (the bony part of your pubic region).
- Strengthen gluteal complex (all three buttocks muscles – maximus, medius and minimus) and stabilise the pelvis through lateral tube walking (i.e. placing band resistance around ankles and stepping sideways – keeping tension on the tube). See exercise #G9.

Exercise

- Avoid any exercise lying on your back (in supine position) after 16 weeks, where gravity is pushing down on the inferior vena cava (large vein), e.g. exercises such as bench press, or prolonged floor work.
- Keep exercise intensity light: low weights, 12-15 repetitions of multiple groups. Some experts feel that using machines in preference to free weights may be more beneficial in the second and third trimester (T1 and T2).
- Overhead movements e.g. shoulder presses should be avoided especially during T3 due to a possible decrease in blood flow to the baby and possible hypertension issues.
- Sudden movements or actions involving position changes – for example, sit to stand, brisk walking, turning and coughing – can cause muscle fibres to spasm resulting in sharp pain felt in one or both sides of the lower abdomen. This pain can last up to 20 minutes and can be alarming. Abdominal bracing or tucking your bottom under (posterior pelvic tilt) may be useful – but seek medical advice if the pain does not subside.
- Decrease or cease rectus abdominus (upper abdominal work, e.g. crunches) and dynamic oblique (waist area) work after T1, especially if diastasis recti occurs (separation of the rectus, which occurs in more than 30% of women).
- Focus on strengthening the pelvic floor and core muscles instead, as these have a huge role to play in the birth and post labour recovery. This really depends on the individual's history of exercise. In my experience working with clients pre-pregnancy on the Swiss ball makes them stronger and more able to exercise during T3.

Hormonal changes

Relaxin is a hormone produced by the ovaries and the placenta, in preparation for childbirth; it relaxes the ligaments in the pelvis, softens and widens the cervix. During pregnancy, relaxin levels are at their highest in T1.

- Avoid lunges in later pregnancy, one leg squats, high step ups and wide squats (lower body unilateral work).

- Many pregnant women may experience "Round Ligament Pain" at some point in their pregnancy. The round ligaments are two fibro muscular cords that extend from the upper portion of the uterus to the labia majora and support the growing uterus.

Stretching

As the baby grows, a woman's abdominal muscles stretch to accommodate the expanding womb, and the extra room needed for this has to come from somewhere. Because the abdominal muscles are stretched far beyond their normal state during pregnancy, they lose their ability to perform their normal role in maintaining body posture. As a result, the lower back takes on an abnormal amount of weight from the torso. Over time, if left untreated, tight muscles will pull on your joints causing postural imbalances and potentially serious pain. Doing the stretches in Group F *Stretching During Pregnancy* will help correct your posture and keep you pain free.

Mobility and Stability Training

The benefit of having a stable pelvis will assist you in performing your exercises with ease. You will enjoy your resistance training, as you have worked on getting these muscles strong. As we covered in the pre-pregnancy section, these two elements are vital in your training, because you will bring your body into balance.

Self-Myofascial Release

This book may be the first time you have heard about myofascial treatment during pregnancy. We will only be using a foam roller and it is important to pay special attention to the instructions. There are certain spots in the body where pressure should not be applied, e.g. glutes area/tailbone area, as this can induce labour. The areas that I suggest for you are safe and effective. As we learned earlier, performing myofascial release helps to release tight spasms (e.g. side of the thigh). It's similar to when your hands are so cold that you can't move your fingers, and after you run them under warm water, they soon become warm and movable again.

Risk of impact injuries

Because an extreme blow or falling on the abdomen can damage the placenta at any stage during pregnancy, avoid activities that may increase the risk of falls such as skiing, ice-skating or those that can result in excessive joint stress such as tennis and other organised sports. Most medical experts agree that the kinds of falls and direct contact that typically occur during contact sports are unlikely to damage either the womb or the baby. Later in pregnancy, the baby moves higher in the womb as it grows and the pelvis no longer protects it as it did in the earlier stages. Consequently, direct impact during sports poses a greater risk of injury to your unborn child at this stage. Because the potential for injury exists, deciding which sports are safe is ultimately up to you and your doctor.

CHAPTER 7

YOUR FITNESS PROGRAM AFTER PREGNANCY

O ne of the dangers of resuming exercise too soon after delivery is that women rush back to the gym before their body is ready. Exercising too soon can cause complications or injuries leading to possible further delays in resuming a normal fitness routine.

Sometimes the fear of injury through doing the wrong exercise prevents some women from beginning exercise; instead, they choose to wait until they have more time or are not as tired. However, doing no exercise after your baby is born can be detrimental to your emotional and physical wellbeing. Issues such as a weak pelvic floor, post natal depression, prolapsed uterus and poor self-image can result. It is so important to take care of yourself all the time but most especially post-pregnancy, as your body goes through some dramatic changes; a bit of applied understanding can mean the difference between a happy healthy and confident you or an unhappy and depressed you.

Different countries, cities and birthing centres would have different protocols in respect to which exercises you are given immediately after the birth. Generally speaking, most hospitals, nursing staff or midwives would encourage you to do pelvic floor muscle contractions, commonly known as Kegel exercises, within days of your delivery. You may feel like you have just run a marathon, after enduring hard and long labour, and the last thing on your mind would be to do any more laboured work – despite the fact that it would benefit you.

You can do something gentle every day following the birth of your baby, even if it's for only few minutes – even as early as the first day after delivery, regardless of whether you had a natural birth or C-section. *Table 8: Ladies' Summarised Training Program – After Pregnancy without any complications – 0-4 weeks* and *Table 9: Ladies' Summarised Training Program – After Pregnancy without any complications – 4-8 weeks* outlines what you can do after delivery. For complicated births, please follow the instructions of your medical support team and your hospital physiotherapist.

A WORD ABOUT YOUR PELVIC FLOOR...

One area where many women struggle or are ignorant but are embarrassed to ask for help or advice, is a weak pelvic floor and decreased satisfaction during intercourse. Your doctor will tell you to begin gentle pelvic floor strengthening exercises straight after your baby is born.

It is important to do these pelvic floor exercises correctly and on a daily basis, which is why I have included specific pelvic floor exercises for you that you may not get from your doctor or gym class. I see many women who are unsure of the anatomy of their pelvic floor and how much to contract these muscles. You can use the information in this book or check with your doctor at your 6 week post-delivery check-up. Your doctor will also advise you when you are ready to resume intercourse with your partner.

Occasionally, women need to see a pelvic floor specialist. Sometimes these muscles can go into spasm and need to be released. Generally speaking, you may only need a couple of treatments. It's always better to address these issues straight away and not try to struggle on without help. The benefits mean that and you will feel encouraged and much better with exercise or sexually with your partner.

No matter how difficult it may be, or how tired you feel, it is worth gathering every ounce of energy to do these exercises. When you do, these exercises will not only have the benefit of preventing poor bladder control (incontinence) and a flatter tummy, but more importantly the improved muscle tone in the pelvic region will give you and your partner greater sexual pleasure and satisfaction.

In some cases, mothers need to see the hospital physiotherapist if there have been unusual tears in muscles or other pelvic floor issues created during pregnancy and/or labour.

Post-delivery, some women will experience sacroiliac joint pain (tailbone area), and/or sciatic nerve related pain. This can also radiate to the lower back and down the side of the leg/hamstring. This calls for a visit to your physiotherapist or chiropractor, as you may need adjustment in your spine before you start exercising.

If an epidural was administered during labour, some women can experience lower back issues for quite some time. So speak to your doctor first and get an understanding of where your body is at and what should be your first choice of treatment.

HOW SOON CAN I BEGIN EXERCISE AFTER THE BIRTH?

Following the birth, many women are extremely eager to get back to their flat tummy and pre-pregnancy shape through exercises like crunches, however I do not advise this course of action. Beside the fact that there are so many other safer options than abdominal crunches, my first recommendation is to work with your medical support staff.

The purpose of your 6 weeks post-delivery check-up is so your doctor can determine whether your body is recovering properly and able to nurture your baby.

As we saw earlier, moderate exercise during lactation does not affect the quantity or composition of breast milk or impact infant growth.[35]

During your 6 week check-up, your doctor should also advise you if you are ready for exercise and also the type of exercise suitable for you, especially post caesarean delivery. During a caesarean delivery, your doctor cuts through four layers of muscles. These muscles need significant time to heal, so please pay particular attention to your doctor's advice on how soon you should begin your exercise regime.

If diabetes or high blood pressure has been a concern during pregnancy, this is an excellent time to address any necessary lifestyle changes and make a commitment to becoming fitter and healthier you.

Post-natal exercises should be chosen with caution. Be selective with the safety of the exercise as well as where you are in terms of post-delivery recovery. There is a degree to which you must assess your own

---

35 Davies, Wolfe, Mottola and MacKinnon in a reprint and modified article from the Canadian Society for Exercise Physiology

individual situation, taking into account pre pregnancy activity, your pregnancy – how active and what kind of exercise you did, as well as the delivery – natural or caesarean, one baby or a multiple birth - consider your set of circumstances.

If lower back pain is an issue, it may be due to various factors; however in most cases it is because not enough attention has been paid to strengthening the pelvic floor and deep abdominal muscles (core) prior to and during pregnancy.

My recommendations for exercising post-delivery, especially in the first 6 weeks, are somewhat conservative. There is certainly a need for pelvic floor and midsection exercises on daily basis. Start with gentle therapeutic exercises such as stretching for 10 minutes a day, or some mobility exercises to loosen up the lower back. See Group B *Stretching Exercises Before and After Pregnancy* and Group C *Mobility and Stability for Before and After Pregnancy – The Secret to a Strong and Stable Pelvis* for more details.

Before you embark on your exercise regime however, make sure you do the "Rectus Abdominal Separation test" below. If you are not sure if you have done this correctly, please consult your physiotherapist or doctor for an accurate assessment.

RECTUS ABDOMINAL SEPARATION TEST.

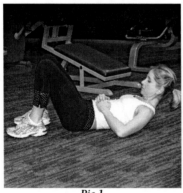 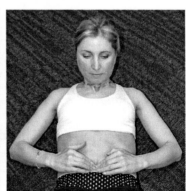

Pic 1   Pic 2

During your pregnancy your rectus abdominals (the 6-pack muscles) separate to make room for the growing baby. This is called rectus abdominal separation or "diastasis recti".

This separation can affect the stability of the torso and can contribute to pelvic floor dysfunction, back and pelvic pain during pregnancy and post-delivery.

You should speak to your obstetrician within few days after delivery to test your rectus abdominals separation. If you have missed this – even at the 6 week check-up, see a physiotherapist to test you.

The level of abdominal separation will vary from woman to woman, the number of pregnancies she has had and how much or how little focus has gone into core stability with each pregnancy.

This separation is measured in the midline/belly button area of your abdomen. If you have 2 to 2.5 fingers separation it is considered problematic. So this is important to you, because the result will determine what abdominal exercises you should start with.

If your separation is in the problematic range, you will need to concentrate on strengthening your pelvic floor and core muscles (i.e. transverse abdominals – corset muscles). Doing crunches will not help you bring the separation any closer, in fact every time you perform a crunch, you are likely to cause more problems as you are strengthening the wrong muscles. Your lower back muscles are likely to be stiff and sore and will not like the movement at all. You need to strengthen the back muscles as well as your core muscles instead of just crunching.

Something that always distresses me is seeing women who have just delivered being instructed to do crunches.

Here is a safe way to test your abdominal separation:

1. Lie on your back with both knees bent and feet hip-width apart.

2. Place both hands at the belly button position (as in pic 2).

3. **Slowly** perform a crunch (as in pic 1) – you should now feel the separation.

4. Remove one hand after you have identified the separation. Use one hand, move your fingertips back and forth across the mid-line of your abdominals.

Normal separation is 1-2 fingers.

If you have more than 2 fingers separation, then you need to do a lot of exercise to build deep abdominal stability. Choose exercises such as the blood pressure cuff (#H19) and 4 point kneeling (#H2, #H3, #H4, and #H5 – choose one for your level).

WHAT EXERCISES ARE SAFE FOR AFTER PREGNANCY?

In the Program Charts, I have suggestions for gentle, therapeutic and deep abdominal/pelvic floor work that are great to begin with for the first 1-8 weeks.

I have 3 programs for the first 3 months after delivery. In these programs you can add cardiovascular exercises such as walking and gentle strengthening work that will cover a total body workout, so that you feel invigorated, happy and healthy. Low impact aerobic classes are terrific for this period. This is NOT the time to hit your maximum heart rate during a treadmill run or to do as many push-ups as you can to test your strength. The goal is to get back in shape, safely and confidently.

From 3 months to 6 months after pregnancy, I have included an additional 3 programs that you can enjoy during the week. If you exercised before and during pregnancy, you can challenge yourself with your resistance training.

Whatever stage you are at post-delivery, there is a program for you. Be sure to choose what is appropriate for you at your stage.

**TABLE 8: LADIES' SUMMARISED TRAINING PROGRAM – AFTER
PREGNANCY WITHOUT ANY COMPLICATIONS – 0-4 WEEKS**

Fitness Program	0-4 weeks	Frequency	Intensity	Time	Type
Cardiovascular	Nil	Nil	Nil	Nil	Nil
Resistance Training	Absolutely NIL *				
Flexibility	Stretches at home	Daily	Low	10-20 mins	Body only, on the Swiss ball
Core/ Abdominal/ Pelvic Floor	At home, floor work A MUST!	Daily	Low	As often as you can	Pelvic floor and stability work

* The only suggestion I would make here is 4 point kneeling, breathing exercise, or the blood pressure intra-abdominal pressure. This should be sufficient to do on a daily basis for the next 4 weeks.

Depending on whether you have a Caesarean section or natural birth will determine what exercises you are able to do immediately' after the birth of your baby.

In a perfect world, it would be a natural birth, preferably with no epidural and then you can start gentle walking and stretches within few weeks of the birth. Ideally, a new mother should sleep, rest and recover for a good 4 to 6 weeks rather than rushing to get back into shape. You will need every ounce of energy for milk production and for your natural flow of hormones to cope with sleepless nights and night feeds.

If you fall into the 35 plus age group, your stamina may not be that of a younger mum, so ***rest is more important than any kind of exercise.***

With Caesareans, doctors cut through 3 layers of muscles, therefore time and rest for healing and getting back on your feet is essential. With this, you will really need to follow your doctor's instructions. You have the rest of your life to get fit and in shape again, it's more important that your healing is accelerated by rest and good, sound nutrition which also helps avoid other complications further along, especially once you re-commence exercise.

In the 'olden' days (and still in some cultures), it was customary for a young mum who had just given birth to go to her mother's house for at least a week and grandmother would help attend to the baby. This was so that the new mum had time to completely recover after enduring her labour (it's almost like running a marathon!). Today, some cultures even practice that it must be at least 2 years before having another baby, as it takes that long for the body to return to normal strength – for the musculoskeletal system to be ready to carry another baby and also to regain a healthy hormonal balance.

So do not rush back into exercise. Take your time, do gentle pelvic floor contractions and exercises such as the *Breathing 4-point Kneeling #H2* which is a great way to start. Every "body" is going to be different, so check with your doctor for advice on when you are ready to do simple and effective exercise. Again I am using 2 weeks as guide, not as a measure of your fitness or any clinical study. If you are really hungry for exercise, then do mainly stretches for the lower back, hips and chest area, or enjoy a gentle stroll with the pram for some fresh air and to get you outdoors.

For a natural birth (with or without epidural), even within the first 24 hours while your uterus is still contracting and shrinking, try to do some gentle pelvic floor contractions. Do not be concerned with the wobbly layer on your tummy! As frightening as it may look, it will recede. I remember having one of those loose and alarming layers of fat and skin that I pinched and extended out, much to my husband's horror! Don't panic! Just give yourself a bit of time and start from the inside with the pelvic floor contractions. This will help you greatly to strengthen ligaments internally in your pelvis and help relieve lower back pain. It will also help your hormonal highs and lows to level out. Remember it will take time.

I see many mothers in the gym who have a great "2-pack" but a bulge below their navel. It does not look good. Many of them will continue doing multiple abdominal crunches but forget about the lower abdominals. Save yourself from the bulge below, and start with the deep abdominal wall – transverse and pelvic floor muscles.

Also worth remembering is that as the transverse abdominals work, it massages your bowels, so if constipation is an issue, this is another way of assisting the bowels to work effectively.

TABLE 9: LADIES' SUMMARISED TRAINING PROGRAM – AFTER PREGNANCY WITHOUT ANY COMPLICATIONS – 4-8 WEEKS

Fitness Program	4-8 weeks	Frequency	Intensity	Time	Type
Cardiovascular	Within 4-6 weeks	3-4 times per week	Light	20-30 mins	Walk, bike or swim
Resistance Training	Light stability work from 6 weeks onwards	3-4 times per week	Light	30 mins	Ball or floor stability work or Yoga
Flexibility	Yes	Daily	Light	20-30 mins	Body only or Yoga
Core, Abdominal, Pelvic floor	Yes	Daily	Light	As often as you can	Floor or ball work

- Caesarean births – please follow your doctor's instructions.
- Births with complications – wait until your 6-8-week post-delivery check-up and follow the guidance of your medical practitioner or physiotherapist.

CHAPTER 8

PELVIC FLOOR MUSCLES

As a young mother, nobody talked to me about pelvic strength before or after the birth of my girls. In my 20 years of experience in the fitness industry, we always concentrated on weight loss, looking great and feeling fantastic. No one was concerned with what muscular imbalances a woman creates by doing the wrong exercises – as long as we looked good!

Is it any wonder women are suffering with incontinence? Every time I taught an aerobics class, I would have a mother tell me how weak her pelvic floor muscles had become since having her baby or subsequent children. What's also sad is that many aerobics instructors have weak pelvic floor muscles due to teaching too many classes well into their third trimester (T3).

This problem may also be due to the presence of the hormone progesterone which causes the muscles and the ligaments to relax and prepare for delivery.

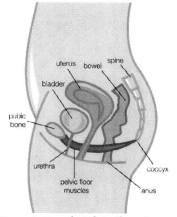

Figure 1: Female Pelvic Floor Anatomy[36]

I cannot stress strongly enough the importance of doing your pelvic floor work. Please understand that it's not "doom and gloom"- you can

---

36 Image courtesy of the Continence Foundation of Australia

get these "unseen" muscles back into shape. You can gain strength and tone in your pelvic floor in as little as 6 weeks if you are committed to train these muscles consistently. Remember, the added benefit also means that your partner will enjoy you more sexually when your pelvic floor muscles are toned, and emotionally you will feel that you are back to your normal sexy self.

When 'lifting' your pelvic floor muscles, make sure you only have a maximum of 20% contraction. Contracting more than that, you will lose the effectiveness and coordination with your lower abdominal muscles. Over-activation of the pelvic floor muscles is not advisable.

Think about all the things you would love to be able to do with your kids like play running with a pram, tennis or snow skiing, but find you just don't have the energy for. Now think about how good you would feel and how it would add so much happiness to you and your family's life if you could do something to change that – to make that dream a reality. Well, the good news is, YOU CAN! Exercise and lifestyle changes begin with you and are the pathway to health and enjoyment in life.

Let's get cracking!

EXERCISE A

SELF–MYOFASCIAL RELEASE (MUSCLE SPASM RELEASE) BEFORE AND AFTER PREGNANCY

The release of muscle spasms will cause some initial discomfort, however if you keep the pressure on a scale of 7/10, the muscle will release (*1 is no pain and 10 is the highest pain threshold*). In most people the iliotibial band (ITB) – the long fibrous tissue on the side of each thigh, glutes/hips, latissimus dorsi (long back muscles) and calves – tends to be tight and requires pressure to release the spasms.

In my experience with clients, practicing the self-myofascial release prior to a cardio or weights program, assists with the mobility of a muscle or joint. In other words, as the muscle releases the tightness, it is not pulling on a joint - hence a movement becomes more fluid instead of restrictive and painful.

For example, as a runner you may find your knees or hips can become sore or stiff. Releasing the trigger points in the ITB (side of the leg), glutes and calves before you go for a run, will make your run a lot easier and you will be able to run with better form, run further and generally feel free in the knees and hips.

To begin with, I recommend 10 minutes of foam roller exercises *before* commencing any cardio, warm up exercises or weight training, and progressively you should only need to release spasms as needed.

Perform the following "muscle spasm releases" *before* cardio or weight training exercises. Choose the most appropriate exercises for you, followed by a stretch for that area. If there is more than one stretch (e.g. for neck), choose one that will work for you. You should aim to do "muscle spasm release" and quick stretches just prior to each workout for a maximum of 5 to 10 minutes.

#A1

NECK RELEASE

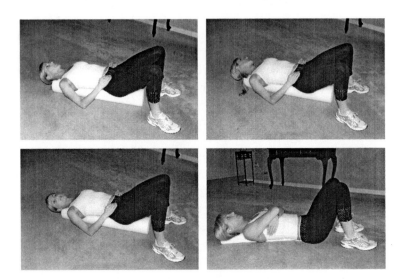

Muscles targeted: Base of the skull, levator scapulae and upper traps *(neck and shoulder muscles).*

Intensity: 5/10

Sets: 1 **Reps:** 2 **Hold:** 10 seconds, followed by neck stretches #B1-B5

1. Place the foam roller from the base of your skull, running in line with your spine, all the way down to your tailbone. Make sure it sits right at the base of the skull, and not on your neck vertebrae. Hands on hips, knees bent and feet slightly wider than hips. You should feel mild pressure into the muscles. Hold that position for 10 seconds.

2. Breathe in; as you breathe out slowly turn your head to one side, now feeling the tension on that same side. Hold that position for

10 seconds. Return to starting position looking up towards the ceiling.

3. Breathing in a normal pattern, turn your head to the opposite side. Hold that position for 10 seconds.

4. You can repeat this few times, usually 2 lots of 10 second holds should be sufficient, however if you feel you need more time on the foam roller and you feel quite comfortable then it's fine to repeat it few times.

Tip:

You may need to vary the position of your head on the foam roller, as there may be some tender spots - pain intensity must not exceed 7/10.

Caution!

If you have a history of neck problems, please see your physiotherapist or osteopath before doing this release.

#A2

LATISSIMUS DORSI

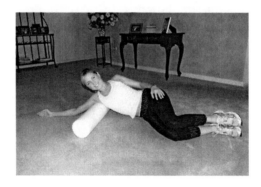

Muscles targeted: Latissimus dorsi (large back muscle).

Intensity: 7/10

Sets: 1 **Reps:** 2 **Hold:** 10 seconds, followed by back stretch
#B6, B7 and B8

1. Position yourself over the foam roller diagonally, so that you are lying totally on your side. The foam roller should be supporting from the armpit to the back of the shoulder blade. You may need to roll yourself forward or backward in order to get into the correct position.

2. Hold that position and tension for 10 to 20 seconds, making sure you are not getting numbness around the shoulder or in your arm.

3. Roll yourself up or down and see if there are any more trigger points to release and repeat the process.

Tip:

Releasing the latissimus dorsi may help you perform exercises such as push-ups and shoulder exercises a lot better.

Your latissimus dorsi and its opposite buttock work together, so make sure you release and strengthen both muscles.

Caution!

If you have any shoulder issues from the past it is best to have them checked before beginning on the foam roller. Releasing muscle spasms around the small tight muscles under the shoulder or around the shoulder blade will be helpful. However any nerve impingement or unstable shoulder needs to be assessed and treated by a physiotherapist or chiropractor.

#A3

RHOMBOIDS

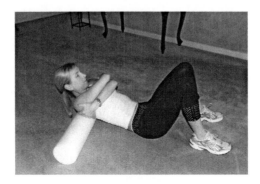

Muscles targeted: Rhomboids
(upper mid back- between shoulder blades).

Intensity: 7/10

Sets: 2 **Reps:** 1 **Hold:** 10 seconds, followed by back stretch #B9

1. Lie on the floor comfortably, with foam roller just below shoulder level. Give yourself a hug and wrap both hands around your shoulders. If you are not able to feel anything, lift your hips off the floor.

2. Roll your upper body to the right side and feel the tension between your spine and shoulder blade. Hold that position for 10 seconds and release.

3. Follow with the left side.

#A4

LOWER BACK

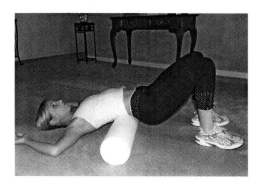

Muscles targeted: Erector spinae
(lower back muscles and abdominals).

Intensity: 6/10

Sets: 2 **Reps:** 1 **Hold:** 20 seconds, followed by lower back stretch #B8,
B11, B12, and B10

1. Lie on the floor with feet slightly further apart than your hips. Lift your hips up and place the foam roller in the small of your back, directly under your belly button. This will help you with creating that curvature in your back, stretching your tummy muscles. If you drop your hip to the right side you will feel the right lower back being released. Hold that tension for 10 – 15 seconds.

2. Repeat on the other side.

3. Taking your arms up, bend the elbows at 90 degrees (as shown). This will give your chest muscles a great stretch at the same time.

Tip:

Notice I have you holding this for a good 20 seconds. This is important because the majority of us have a rounded upper back. Also, our lower back generally slouches with prolonged periods of time sitting at a desk.

#A5

HIPS AND ITB

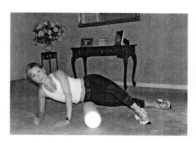 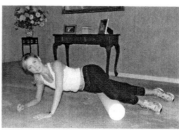

Muscles targeted: Hips and ITB (iliotibial band - thin layer of muscle fascia on side of leg).

Intensity: 7/10

Sets: 2 **Reps:** 1 **Hold:** 15 seconds, followed by hip stretches #B13 and B10

The release of tightness in the hip and ITB makes an enormous difference in walking, running, squatting and performing daily activities. Some people are very tight and may find it a challenge to hold the pressure for even 10 seconds, but others may find it comfortable. Whatever category you are in, stay within your comfort zone and progressively release the tightness, instead of feeling too sore and giving up.

1. Lie on the foam roller sideways on your right hip. Support yourself on your right forearm and use your left arm in front the body to stabilise. You may need to hold that position for more than 15 seconds, as the muscles around the hips are quite tight.

2. Roll the foam roller upwards towards the heart, as there may be another trigger point that needs releasing.

3. Next, move away from your hip and now target your ITB, (the band (fascia) that attaches mid-section of your thigh and hamstrings muscles). In this instance, you will need to take care of the front and back of the thigh.

4. Slowly roll yourself up and down on the foam roller at mid-section, until you find a relatively comfortable spot with pain intensity being about 7/10. Hold that position and tension for 10-15 seconds.

5. If you are able to handle the tension, roll to the next tender spot and repeat.

#A6

Buttocks and Piriformis

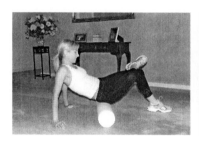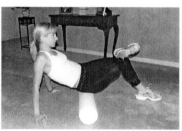

Muscles targeted: All three gluteus muscles and piriformis (deep buttock muscle, where the sciatic nerve runs through).

Intensity: 7/10

Sets: 2 **Reps:** 1 **Hold:** 20 seconds, followed by buttocks stretch #B10

The glute medius (hip muscle) is a tight and weak muscle. If you don't release spasms, stretch and strengthen this muscle, you will not be able to stabilise through your pelvis while doing squats and lunges. It is much the same with the piriformis muscle – I call the piriformis the "pain in the butt" muscle. The sciatic nerve runs through this muscle, so someone with sciatic pain needs to release tension through the piriformis and do nerve stretches in order to get the whole musculature functioning properly.

1. Sit on the foam roller on your right buttock. Support yourself using your arms behind the foam roller.

2. Place your right foot on top of your left knee.

3. Tilt your thighs sideways (on your right buttock) and feel the tension. Hold it for 10-20 seconds. You may roll up or down in order to find the tensest spot in your muscle.

4. Swap to the other side.

5. If you experience one side tighter than the other, repeat that side.

Caution!

Do not do this release during pregnancy as it is too close to the sacrum (tailbone) and will induce labour.

#A7

CALF

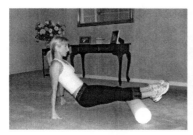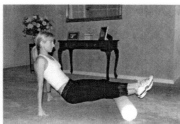

Muscles targeted: Calves.

Intensity: 7/10

Sets: 1 **Reps:** 1 **Hold:** 15 seconds, followed by calf stretch #B15

1. Place the foam roller just below your calves.

2. Support yourself using your arms and lift your buttocks off the floor.

3. Start rolling your calves over the foam roller in a forward motion.

4. Feel the tension and hold that position for 10-15 seconds.

5. You may also test the outside of the calves and, if you find some spasm spots, hold that position for a further 10 seconds.

#A8

SHINS

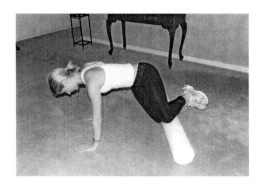

Muscles targeted: Shins.

Intensity: 6/10

Sets: 1 **Reps:** 1 **Hold:** 10 seconds, followed by shin stretch #B16

If you have sore shins you may be better to have them massaged before you attempt the roller, as they can feel quite tender and sore.

1. Supporting most of your body weight using your arms, place the foam roller just below your knees on the side of shin.

2. Shift your body weight to one side, until you feel the tension in your shin.

3. Hold that position for 10 seconds, and further roll yourself up until you find another tender spot and hold again for 10 seconds.

4. Swap to the other side.

#A9

FRONT THIGH

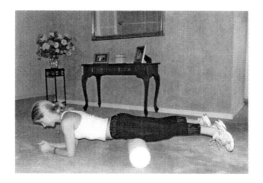

Muscles targeted: Hips and rectus femoris (middle thigh muscle).

Intensity: 6/10

Sets: 1 **Reps:** 1 **Hold:** 15 seconds, followed by hip and thigh stretch #B13 and B14

1. Lie on the foam roller on the front of your thighs.

2. Start just below the hip level and work your way down.

3. You may experience different tight and tender spots on each leg, nevertheless continue releasing and it should balance out. The pain scale around the front of the hip is mild, so experiencing 6/10 pain scale will be as much as you can get.

4. Hold that position for 10-15 seconds before moving on to another.

Exercise B

Stretching Exercises Before and After Pregnancy

Chapter 3 "Your Fitness Program Before Pregnancy", outlined the reasons why stretching is such an important part of your exercise program. In the following pages, you will find a good outline of stretches for before and after pregnancy. Please note however, that stretches for during pregnancy are in a separate chapter because your body is going through different hormonal changes. (Stretching during pregnancy is recommended but not at the same level or intensity).

You have probably heard the phrase "An ounce of prevention is worth a pound of cure"; this is certainly the case with stretching. Do not cheat yourself by thinking "I'll be fine!"

Using the Contract-relax method in your stretching will benefit you greatly, as the muscles relax and are more effectively mobilised.

Contract-relax stretch is a method where a muscle is placed under tension, without movement of the proximal (close) joint. Breathing through a Contract-relax stretch focuses you on your breathing, thereby increasing the value of the stretch. Holding the breath during a 5-count contract phase allows the muscle to go through tension, therefore when you breathe out, the release from tension allows the muscle greater stretch.

#B1

NECK – BACK

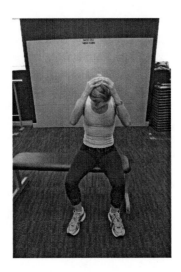

Muscles targeted: Neck, skull and mid-back.

Sets: 1 **Reps:** 1 **Hold:** 20 seconds

1. Sit up tall on a bench with your neck relaxed, looking straight ahead.

2. Breathe in; as you breathe out, gently drop your chin towards your chest. Hold and relax.

3. Place both hands on top of your head. Do not pull.

Tip:

The purpose of this stretch is to release tension and increase mobility. For a better stretch, you may use the contract-relax method. Breathe in and as you breathe out, push your head back into your hands with a mild pressure. Hold that pressure for 5 seconds. Repeat this 2-3 times.

#B2

NECK – SIDE

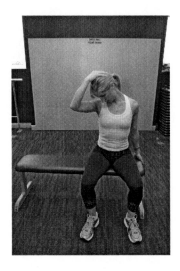

Muscles targeted: Upper trapezius (base of skull and neck muscles).

Sets: 1 **Reps:** 1 **Hold:** 10 seconds

1. Sit up with a tall posture on a bench, with one hand behind holding on the bench anchoring the shoulder down and the other gently placed on top of head.

2. Breathe in and as you breathe out, turn your chin down toward your armpit.

3. Breathe in again, and as you breathe out feel the neck relax further down.

4. Repeat other side.

Tip:

For a greater stretch, perform a Contract-relax stretch by gently pushing your head up while your hand is resisting the tension. Hold the pressure for 5 seconds. As you release the stretch, you should feel the neck gain more flexibility. Release and you may repeat this for 2-3 times. Repeat other side.

#B3

NECK– FRONT

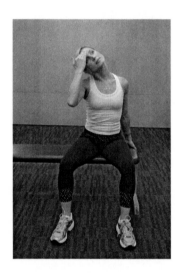

Muscles targeted: Neck-scalenes (deep front of neck muscles).

Sets: 1 Reps: 1 Hold: 10 seconds

1. Sit tall on a bench, anchor the shoulder with one hand behind holding on the bench.

2. Turn your head to the side and lift your chin towards the ceiling as if you are tilting your head backwards. Place your fingers against the forehead.

3. Breathe in; as you breathe out gently push your forehead into your hands and hold that tension for 5 seconds.

4. As you release the stretch, you should feel the front and side of your neck gain more flexibility. Release and repeat 2-3 times.

5.   Repeat the other side.

Tip:

Stretches for the side and front of the neck also help with diaphragmatic breathing. This stretch will also help release tension from the first rib under your clavicle. This means your push-ups will improve in quality.

#B4

NECK – SIDE

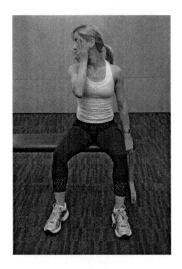

Muscles targeted: Side of neck.

Sets: 1 **Reps:** 1 **Hold:** 10 seconds

1. Sit tall on a bench and turn your head looking over your right shoulder. Take the opposite hand (left) to your cheek and just hold to a comfortable but noticeable stretch.

2. Breathe in; as you breathe out, gently create tension with your head pressing against your hand and hold for 5 seconds.

3. Release and repeat 2-3 times.

4. Repeat the other side.

Tip:

Do not strain or press too hard, the aim is to release tension, not lock up the neck.

#B5

NECK – BACK

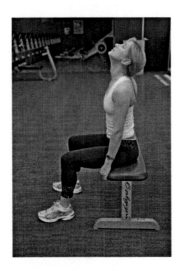

Muscles targeted: Front of neck.

Sets: 1 **Reps:** 1 **Hold:** 10 seconds

1. Sit up tall on a bench and look straight ahead.

2. Breathe in; as you breathe out, gently tilt your head backwards feeling the front of the neck open up. Hold that position for 10-15 seconds.

3. Breathe in with your head still in a stretched position, and then as you come back up, breathe out.

4. Repeat 2-3 times.

Tip:

If you want to increase the stretch in the front of your neck, swallow and place your tongue on the roof of your mouth. Then gently tilt your head back as far as you are comfortable. Return to your starting position.

#B6

UPPER BACK

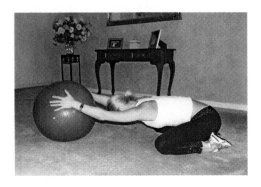

Muscles targeted: Latissimus dorsi, back and arms.

Sets: 1 **Reps:** 1 **Hold:** 10-20 seconds

1. Taking a Swiss ball, kneel on the floor comfortably, placing both hands on top of the ball. You can easily relax in this position or slowly and gently push the ball away from you, allowing the side of your back to stretch.

2. To intensify the stretch, roll the ball from one side to the other feeling the stretch from your hips through to your shoulders and arms.

Tip:

If you do not have a Swiss ball, you can perform the stretch against the wall.

#B7

UPPER BACK

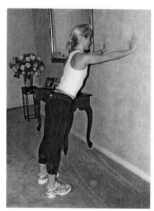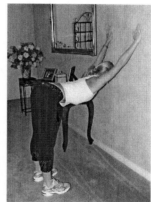

Muscles targeted: Latissimus dorsi, back and arms.

Sets: 1 **Reps:** 1 **Hold:** 10 seconds

The beauty of this stretch on the wall is that you can get a lovely hamstring stretch at the same time.

1. Place straight arms with palms on the wall at eye level.

2. Relax your upper body and shoulders and take a deep breath in.

3. As you are breathing out, gently allow your upper body to fall down towards the floor, feeling the stretch in your arms, chest, upper back behind the arms and lower back.

4. If you are not comfortable with the hamstrings being stretched, you may bend your knees slightly. However, the more you do this stretch the easier it will become and you will enjoy it more.

5. Hold this position for 10-20 seconds or simply repeat it a few times, each time allowing your body to relax and stretch further.

#B8

LOWER BACK

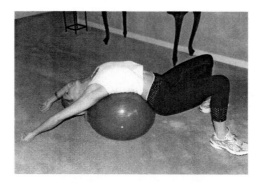

Muscles targeted: Lower back, upper back, abdominals and chest.

Sets: 1 Reps: 1 Hold: 10 seconds

This is an excellent stretch for the lower back, as most of us are either in a sitting or standing position throughout the day.

1. Lie on a Swiss ball wrapping your lower back around the ball/

2. If you are comfortable in this position, extend your arms overhead and feel the chest open up.

3. You can hold this as long as you wish or as is comfortable.

4. Feel free to repeat this stretch if you find it relaxing.

Tip:

To reverse a daily rounded posture, stretch the abdominal area. Open the chest, abdominal area and ribcage. Your abdominal wall needs stretching also, particularly if you are accustomed to doing too many crunches.

#B9

LOWER BACK

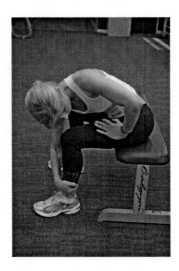

Muscles targeted: Lower back, hips and ITB (Iliotibial band).

Sets: 2-3 **Reps:** 1 **Hold:** 10 seconds

This stretch has a different approach, as it is from a seated position, and targets the upper back and shoulder as well as the lower back.

1. Sit on a bench or a chair with feet wider than shoulder-width apart. Place your left hand on the left thigh.

2. Rotate your body half way to the left side.

3. Slowly bend forward and towards the left knee, so that your trunk is hanging over the thigh. Your right hand is wrapped around the outside of your left ankle.

4. Breathe in; as you breathe out, create a rounded curvature in your upper back, then gently pull away from your left thigh. Maintain your curve and hold for 10-15 seconds.

5. Repeat the stretch 2-3 times, swapping over to the other side each time. Rest up to 30 seconds between each set.

#B10

LOWER BACK

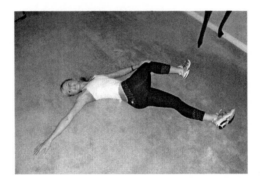

Muscles targeted: Lower back, glutes, hips and ITB.

Sets: 1 **Reps:** 1 **Hold:** 20 seconds

1. Lie on your back with right arm extended and right leg across the body.

2. Keep your right shoulder on the floor during the stretch.

3. Keep your extended leg straight, although soft at the knee, and feel your body nice and long.

4. Place your left hand on the outside of your right knee and gently press down. Breathing is very important in this position, so during your 20 seconds stretch take deep breaths in and out. By doing this, your lower back and hips will relax into a more enjoyable stretch.

Tips:

If you feel there is some locking or stiffness in your upper or lower back, or outside or inside hip, make sure you see your physiotherapist or osteopath to adjust vertebrae or muscle tissue.

Everyone has different flexibility and mobility, so make sure you are only taking the leg across as far as you are comfortable.

You may feel a greater stretch using the Contract-relax method. Place the opposite hand on the bent knee and breathe in. As you breathe out gently push against your hand. The pressure should be mild and comfortable. Release the stretch. Repeat the stretch for 2-3 times until you feel you are comfortable with the stretch. Repeat on the other side.

#B11

McKenzie Press-up

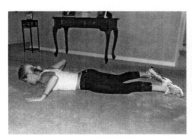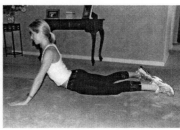

Muscles targeted: Lower back and tummy, and chest.

Sets: 1 **Reps:** 10 **Tempo:** 3:2:3

This stretch is known as the "McKenzie Stretch or Back & Chest Stretch". If you have been unfortunate to have some lower back issues, this is one of the stretches that are very often prescribed as part of a rehabilitation or stretch program.

1. Lie on your stomach with your arms and hands out to the side, similar to the way you would do a push-up.

2. Breathe in; as you breathe out lift your chest off the floor, leaving your hips in contact with the floor. Be sure that you are not shrugging your shoulders, but instead relax your shoulder blades down towards your hips.

3. Repeat this for 10 repetitions with a tempo of going up for 3 counts, hold it for 2 and release it for 3.

Tips:

As you are coming up and breathing out, you should feel your lower back relaxed and not tensing up.

You may do this in the morning and also last thing at night before you go to sleep, as it will mobilise and release the stiffness in your lower back, thus helping you with better sleep.

#B12

RUSSIAN TWIST

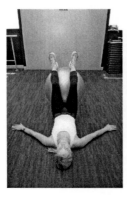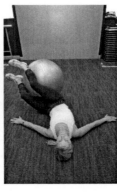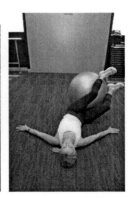

Muscles targeted: Lower back.

Sets: 1 **Reps:** 10 **Tempo:** 3:1:3

This is one of the most effective stretches, as it also works on the core muscles.

1. Lie on your back with the ball placed close to your hamstrings and buttocks with calves on top of ball.

2. Arms are out to the side at forty-five degrees, with palms down for support. Do this stretch and release slowly, in other words allow your lower body to twist only to a point that your shoulders are maintaining floor contact. Breathe in as you breathe out, allow your lower body to slowly fall to the left – thus stretching out the right lower back. Bring the ball back to the middle.

3. Repeat the right side, allowing your left lower back to be stretched.

4. You want to have a tempo of 3:1:3, which is going sideways for 3 counts, hold for 1 count and come up for 3 counts. Repeat the same counting on the other side.

Tip:

To perform a stretch only, do 1 set of 10 repetitions. However it can also be used as a strengthening abdominal exercise with 2-3 sets with 60 seconds rest between each set.

#B13

HIP AND THIGH WITH SWISS BALL

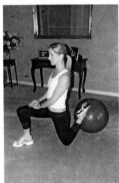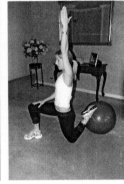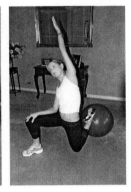

Muscles targeted: Hip flexors, psoas (deep abdominal/hip muscles) and all 4 thigh muscles.

Sets: 2 Reps: 1 Hold: 10 seconds

The hip flexor stretch is one of the most neglected stretches and is sometimes rushed. You must do this stretch on a daily basis as lower back can sometimes become stiff due to the hips being really tight.

If you are in an office environment where sitting for prolonged periods of time is normal, this stretch should become as regular as brushing your teeth.

1. From a kneeling position, place one foot on the top of the ball. The front leg should be well at the front with knee bent at 90 degrees.

2. You should now feel the stretch as it is opening your hip. The quad muscles should feel a greater stretch.

3. To make this stretch more intense, contract your buttocks on the same side that you are stretching your hip. Hold for 5 seconds and release. Repeat it again and hold it for further 5 seconds.

4. To intensify this stretch to include the psoas muscle (deep abdominal muscle from your ribcage to your hip), take one arm up and lengthen it towards the ceiling.

5. Breathe in; as you breathe out lean forward about 10 degrees and reach further with your arm. Hold this position for 10 seconds.

Tip:

If your kneeling knee is experiencing a little discomfort, place a towel or a cushion underneath it to soften the impact.

#B14

HIP AND INNER THIGH

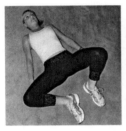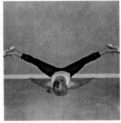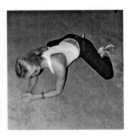

Muscles targeted: Inner thigh.

Sets: 1 **Reps:** 1 **Hold:** 60 seconds

I have three different versions for the inner thigh stretch that I have found beneficial with clients. Try each one of them on different days and see which one best suits you.

1. Lie on your back with both knees bent and feet together. Slowly let both knees open up until your legs can't go any further. You may hold this stretch for up to 5 minutes.

2. *The second version is the wall stretch, which is quite comfortable and can be used while you are pregnant in T1.*

   Lie on the floor with your buttocks positioned close to the wall. Breathing normally, allow both legs to go out and down the wall. When you have reached a comfortable position, you may hold this stretch for up to 5 minutes.

   To come out of the stretch, use your hands if you need assistance with bringing both legs to the starting position.

3. *The third version is from a kneeling position.*

Place both arms and hands on the floor for support. Gently open both knees sideways until you feel a comfortable stretch in your inner thighs. Hold this stretch for 20 seconds.

#B15

CALF

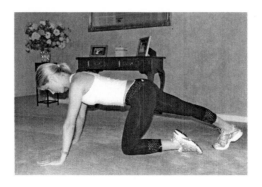

Muscles targeted: Calves.

Sets: 1 **Reps:** 1 **Hold:** 20 seconds

1. From a kneeling position, take one leg back and rest your foot on your toes.

2. Breathe in; as you breathe out, transfer your body weight on the back leg and push your heel backwards until you feel your calf stretching out.

3. Hold that position for 20 seconds. Repeat on the other side.

#B16

SHIN

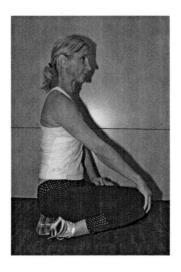

Muscles targeted: Tibia (shins).

Sets: 2 Reps: 1 **Hold:** 10 seconds

This is a very common problem especially for runners and walkers. Chronic shin splints can become very sore and hard to manage. I highly recommend that you follow my program with the foam roller to release the spasms and micro trauma caused by overuse and then follow with this stretch.

1. From a kneeling position, take your right hand – hold and lift your knee away from the floor.

2. Feet should be relaxed under your glutes. You should feel the shin stretch from your ankle all the way to the knee.

3. Your other hand is resting on the opposite thigh. Repeat on the other side.

4. Hold the stretch on each shin for 20 seconds.

Tip:

It's important to stretch the calves and shins in the same session.

#B17

HAMSTRING

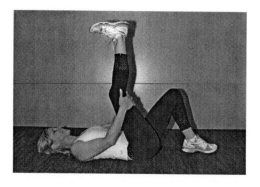

Muscles targeted: Hamstrings.

Sets: 2 **Reps:** 1 **Hold:** 20 seconds

Hamstrings need a lot of attention and stretching. Make sure that you do not overstretch. It's not always the feeling of burn in the stretch that will give you the best result.

1. Lie on your back with both knees bent. Bring one leg up with a slight bend at the knee, holding either your ankle or just behind the knee.

2. Flatten your lower back while you gently bring the leg towards your torso. You may only need to extend or bring your leg to a straight position to feel the stretch.

3. Do not pull your leg so tight as to lift your glutes off the floor. Just bring to about 50% of the maximum tension in your hamstrings.

4. Hold the stretch on each leg for 20 seconds. Repeat on the other side.

Tip:

For greater results, perform a Contract-relax stretch on the hamstring. From the same position, while holding your ankle or behind the knee, place gentle tension on the hamstring as if you are pushing the leg down towards the floor. Hold this for 5 counts, and breathe out when you release it. You will notice the leg will have greater flexibility.

EXERCISE C

MOBILITY AND STABILITY FOR BEFORE AND AFTER PREGNANCY – THE SECRET TO A STRONG AND STABLE PELVIS

I have put together a number of stability exercises and I suggest that you try them all. See which ones you like the most, get the benefits from them and keep practising them. Ultimately, they will all give you results and they are gentle on the body. You will feel yourself getting stronger even if you begin with only one set of exercises each day.

On the program chart I have only 1 set of 10 repetitions however, if you find yourself enjoying the exercises, you can make it a total work-out by doing 2 or 3 sets of 10 repetitions. You can perform each of the stability exercises every day or every second day; there is no particular prescription, as they are very gentle on the body.

You may notice I refer to *tempo of movement,* which means how long you should hold a position. For example, you see a tempo of 3:2:3 on the hip extension floor version exercise - that means, you will lift up for 3 counts, hold that position for 2 counts and lower yourself down for 3 counts.

If I have you holding a certain position for 5 seconds (e.g. 3:5:3), it simply means you are giving that particular muscle a longer contraction - this means you will lift for 3 counts, hold that position for 5 counts, and lower to your starting position for 3 counts.

#C1

HIP EXTENSION FLOOR VERSION

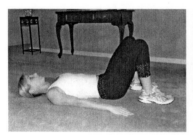 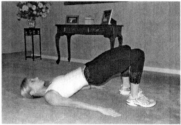

Beginner.

Muscles targeted: Hips, gluteus, hamstrings and lower back.

Sets: 1-3 **Reps:** 10 **Tempo:** 3:2:3 **Rest:** 30 seconds

1. Lie on your back with both knees bent, feet hip-width apart and palms out to 45 degrees.

2. Breathe in; as you breathe out, lift your pelvic floor muscles and contract your lower abdominals by pressing your lower back towards the floor, feeling the tailbone lift off the floor.

3. Start lifting your hips and glutes off the floor for a count of 3, hold it for 2 counts at the top, and lower your hips back down for 3 counts.

4. Maintain the contraction the whole time with your pelvic floor muscles and lower abdominal wall. During this time, try holding the position while squeezing your glutes for a count of 5 for a more intense load.

5. To release the extension start releasing down from mid-back, vertebrae by vertebrae with the tail bone down last. Repeat this 5-10 times for 1-3 sets.

Caution!

Only extend as far as is comfortable, being careful to avoid any lower back pain or pressure. Stop immediately if you experience any pain.

Make sure you are pushing through your heels, and that the glutes are working effectively, feeling your hips open fully.

#C2

HIP EXTENSION FLOOR VERSION – (ALTERNATE LEG)

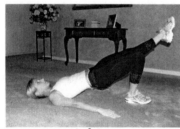 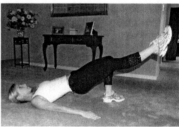

Left Leg   *Right Leg*

Intermediate.

Muscles targeted: Hips, gluteus, hamstrings and lower back.

Sets: 2 **Reps:** 10 **Tempo:** 5 second hold **Rest:** 60 seconds

Progression from Hip Extension (exercise #C1) to alternating leg version means that you will be challenging the glutes and hips more. So, to work on your strength throughout your hips, give this exercise a go. I guarantee that your glutes will feel toned and strong.

1. Bring both feet together, come up to full extension of the hips and progress with extending one leg out. Hold for 5 seconds.

2. Maintain your hip alignment and make sure your pelvis is not dipping to one side. Hold the leg extended for a count of 5.

3. Change to other leg. Repeat this with holding each leg up for 5 counts. Perform total of 10 repetitions – which is 5 lifts on each leg. Have a 60-second break and repeat again without stretching.

Tip:

In this exercise, make sure that both thighs are of equal height and that you are really feeling the glute working i.e. if the right leg is straight – it's the left glute that is working to keep you up and vice versa – therefore creating the stability and strength.

#C3

HIP EXTENSION – SWISS BALL VERSION

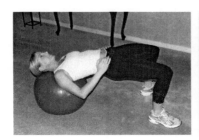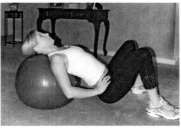

Intermediate.

Muscles targeted: Hips, gluteus, hamstrings and lower back.

Sets: 1-3 **Reps:** 10 **Tempo:** 3:2:3 **Rest:** 60 seconds

Progression from beginner to intermediate level would be from floor version to using a Swiss ball.

1. From a seated position, walk forward with your feet, until you roll yourself on your back. Ensure your head, shoulders and upper back is supported on the ball. Your feet should be comfortably wider than your hips, and both hands on your hips.

2. Lower your hips and glutes to the floor, without your head and shoulders lifting off the ball. Breathe in, and as you breathe out, contract your core muscles while you are down there. Lift your hips and glutes to full extension squeezing the glutes. Perform 1-3 sets.

Tip:

You should not be rolling the ball forward and back, but rather lifting your hips up and down.

#C4

HIP EXTENSION WITH ABDUCTION USING BALL (OUTER THIGH)

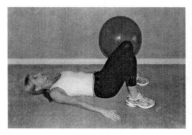 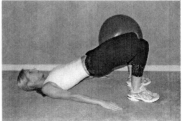

Beginner and Intermediate.

Muscles targeted: Outer thigh, hips, hamstrings and deep abdominal wall.

Sets: 2-3 **Reps:** 10 **Tempo:** 2:2:2 **Rest:** 0-60 seconds

Physiotherapists commonly prescribe this exercise as an easy way to strengthen the hips (glute medius), particularly if there are some knee problems and loading-up on the legs is not advisable.

1. Lie on your back with the ball elevated off the floor against the wall at the knee level (see photo).

2. Connect your deep abdominal wall while maintaining feet at hip-width apart with your arms relaxed at your sides.

3. Without compromising your position and posture, gently lift your hips into a bridge-like position. Push the outside of your knee onto the ball. Hold for 2 seconds, release the push and then gently lower yourself to the floor. Repeat for 10 repetitions and do the other side.

4. This can be done for 2-3 sets of 10 repetitions as a warm up before squatting, before a walk or run or as a strengthening exercise for the glutes and stability for the knee. Rest between each side will depend on your strength. If you are feeling strong then swap sides, if you need rest, then rest up to 60 seconds between each set.

#C5

HIP EXTENSION – ADDUCTION WITH BALL (INNER THIGH)

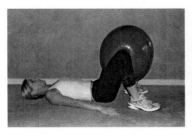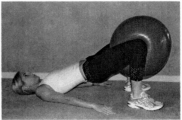

Beginner and Intermediate.

Muscles targeted: Inner thigh, pelvic floor, deep abdominal wall and gluteus.

Sets: 2-3 **Reps:** 10 **Tempo:** 2:2:2 **Rest:** 60 seconds

This exercise can be performed with a towel, medicine ball or a small Swiss ball (as pictured).

Working the inner thigh is just as important as the outer thigh – not just one or the other – as both inner and outer work together – much like the front and back of the thigh.

1. Lie on your back, with the ball or towel between your legs.

2. Connect your deep abdominal muscles together with your pelvic floor, lift your hips up, and squeeze the ball for 2 seconds.

3. The pressure within your inner thighs should be gentle and mild.

4. Maintain gentle pressure in your pelvic floor area, remembering these are weak and will need gradual strengthening.

5. Repeat for 10 repetitions for 2-3 sets. Rest for 60 seconds between each set and perhaps stretch the inner thighs between each set. (This is the only time I will recommend a stretch as the inner thigh never gets sufficient stretching. You will feel the difference in your strength and flexibility in this area once you do this exercise.)

#C6

BASIC 4–POINT KNEELING

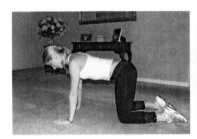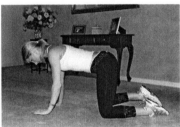

Beginner.

Muscles targeted: Transverse abdominals, (deep abdominal muscle), pelvic floor, multifidus (deep spine muscle) and shoulder stabilisers.

Sets: 1-3 **Reps:** 10 **Tempo:** 10 sec hold **Rest:** 60-120 seconds

1. Position yourself in a 4-point kneeling stance. Make sure your hands are directly under your shoulders and your knees are directly under your hips.

2. Your spine should be nice and long with a natural curvature in the neck and lower back.

3. Relax through your shoulder blades gently pulling them toward your spine then down towards your hips.

4. Take in a nice diaphragmatic breath, similar to when you do a yawn. As you breathe out, (without shifting your hips or pelvis) lift your pelvic floor muscles and draw your bellybutton in towards your spine.

5. You should feel a mild contraction - maintain that for at least 5 counts for beginners, however your target is 10 seconds.

6. Please ensure that you are not over contracting your pelvic floor muscles. In other words, don't contract 100% of your capacity. About 10-20% of your maximum is the correct contraction here. Doing the wrong contraction can cause burnout in that muscle, leading to prolapsed uterus as you age.

7. Repeat this breathing and contraction exercise for as many times as you can. Start with 1 set of 10 contractions. Ideally, 1-3 sets of 10 second holds.

Progression:

When you are able to do 3 sets with good form holding each for 10 seconds, you are able to progress to lifting opposite hand and knee off the floor. Make sure you have 60-120 seconds rest between each set, as this type of exercise requires intense mental focus and therefore can be quite challenging to the neural system.

Tip:

These muscles are similar to the marathon-type muscle fibres, and as such are designed to support the load of your internal organs and your baby. That is why longer mild contractions are recommended.

#C7

4-Point Kneeling With Opposite Arm And Leg Extension

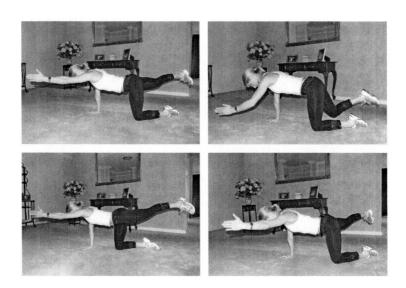

Intermediate.

Muscles targeted: Transverse abdominals, (deep abdominal muscle), pelvic floor, multifidus (deep spine muscle). Latissimus dorsi, shoulder stabilisers and glutes.

Sets: 2-3 **Reps:** 10 **Tempo:** 4:2:4 **Rest:** 60 seconds

This is one of my favourite exercises and it is excellent for creating stability and strength in the midsection.

The impact is nil, and it's a stand-alone exercise that can be done anytime, anywhere.

1. From the basic 4-point kneeling position, progress to taking the opposite arm and opposite leg out simultaneously. Hold that for a comfortable count of 2. Your trunk should not move at all while extending your arm and leg. If you find you are unstable or wobbling, regress to the previous exercise.

2. Do not take your arm and leg out until you have good control and contraction in the pelvic floor and deep abdominal wall, as this will prevent you from being wobbly.

3. Perform as many as you are able, using a tempo of 4 counts out, hold for 2 and 4 counts back in. Your goal should be to complete 2-3 sets of 10 repetitions with 60 seconds rest between each set.

Tip:

If you have discomfort in your hands or knees, go to the blood pressure cuff exercise (#H19). Do not place padding under the knees, as this will alter the hip alignment and the exercises will be faulty.

#C8

SUPERMAN – ALTERNATIVE TO THE FLOOR 4–POINT KNEELING

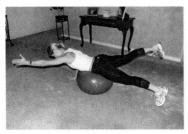 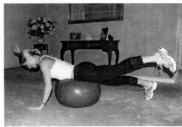

Beginner.

Muscles targeted: Upper back, lower back, gluteus, latissimus dorsi.

Sets: 1-3 **Reps:** 10 **Tempo:** 3:3:3 **Rest:** 30-60 seconds

This is an easier option, however I find that the deep abdominal wall does not connect as much as doing the floor version. Your tummy being on the ball prevents you from contracting the core muscles properly and effectively. You may begin with this version and progress to the floor.

1. Lie on the ball with your tummy in a comfortable position. Same principle applies as the floor using the 4-point kneeling version.

2. When you feel you have stabilised, take one leg and opposite arm out with your hand in a "thumbs-up" position. Hold that position for 2 seconds and make sure your leg is completely straight to ensure your glutes are contracting. The extended leg should not be any higher than the hips or glutes.

3. Repeat from side to side, without sacrificing form. As soon as you feel your technique is suffering, stop the exercise and rest for 60 seconds.

4. Perform 1-3 sets with 10 repetitions in total with a tempo of 3:3:3.

#C9

SINGLE LEG LIFT – ON BALL

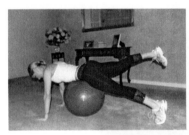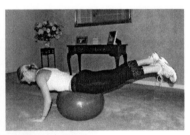

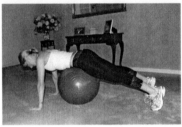

Beginner and Intermediate.

Muscles targeted: Gluteus predominantly (but also hamstrings and lower back).

Sets: 2 Reps: 10 Tempo: 2:2:2 **Rest:** 60 seconds

This exercise can be used for warm up or strengthening. It is more challenging because you are using and unstable object (Swiss Ball).

1. If you are not strong and stable through your glutes, start with single leg version first with 3 sets of 10 with 60 seconds rest between each set. If you are using this exercise as a warm up, complete 2 sets of 10 repetitions with 30 seconds rest.

2. The speed or the tempo for this version is lifting the leg for 2 counts, holding it for 2 counts and lowering for 2 counts, so

you have a nice consistent movement. Make sure that your leg is completely straight and do not bend the knee, otherwise, you will work the hamstring more than the glutes.

3. Lie on your tummy on the ball with a comfortable position and contract your pelvic floor and deep abdominal wall (pull your belly button away from the ball).

4. Lift both legs up in a controlled manner (2 counts up, hold for 2 and 2 counts down) without throwing or bouncing your legs. Keep your legs very straight the entire time as this will avoid the use of hamstrings, concentrating on the glutes. Return to starting position and lift again.

Tip:

Keep the head aligned with the spine. Do not lock your elbows.

#C10

PRONE COBRA – SWISS BALL VERSION

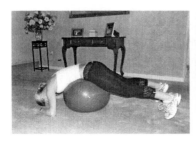 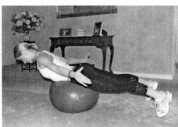

Arms outwards and thumbs upwards

Beginner and Intermediate.

Muscles targeted: Upper back, lower back and gluteus.

Sets: 1-3 **Reps:** 10 **Tempo:** 2:2:2 **Rest:** 60 seconds

1. Lie over the ball with forearms and head relaxed towards the floor. Feet wider than shoulder-width apart, so you stay supported.

2. Breathe in; as you breathe out draw your belly button away from the ball while lifting your pelvic floor muscles.

3. Only then, you may come up with your arms extended at 45 degrees and thumbs up (facing the ceiling). Hold that position for 2 seconds. Breathe in and go down, breathe out and come up.

4. Although this is a nice strengthening exercise for the back, you should also feel a lovely stretch in the chest area.

5. Tempo for this should be up for 2 counts, hold for 2 and release for 2.

Tip:

If you do not have a ball or you are having trouble with the balance, you can perform the same exercise on the floor without the ball. Do not come up too high though. You should not feel any back pain with this.

#C11

LATERAL BALL ROLL

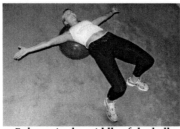

Balance in the middle of the ball

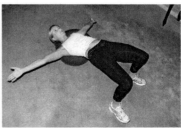

Travel to right, left shoulder blade is on the ball

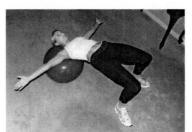

Travel to left, right shoulder blade is on the ball

Intermediate.

Muscles targeted: Hips, gluteus, core and hamstrings.

Sets: 1-2 **Reps:** 8-12 **Tempo:** Slow **Rest:** 60 seconds

This exercise is more suited to the intermediate person who may have trained for some time before falling pregnant and possibly trained during pregnancy under the guidance and supervision of a personal trainer.

1. Lie on the ball with your head and shoulders well supported. Take both arms out to the side, palms facing up and at shoulder height.

2. Before travelling from side to side, ensure that your deep abdominal muscles and pelvic floor are contracted during the movement.

3. With your feet, in a heel-toe-heel-toe movement, travel to the right side until you feel your right glute (predominantly) and leg take the load and balance for 1-2 counts. Return to the beginning and travel to the left side and hold for 1-2 counts.

4. This can be used as a warm up exercise of 1-2 sets of 10 repetitions in total, or as part of your full weights program with 3 sets of 8-12 repetitions with 60 seconds rest between each set.

Tip:

As you travel to each side, lift your head up and slightly tuck your chin in. Have a look at your hips and see that your hips are level without one side dipping. If this is the case, regress your lateral travel and lift up the side that is dipping so that the glutes are working effectively. Keep your chin tucked in during the travel period.

Exercise D

Strengthening Exercises for Before and After Pregnancy

The challenge when purchasing a book and following an exercise program is that one person may be at one fitness level and another person may be at a completely different level with various body shapes and statistics.

To make things simple and easy to follow, we will gauge your level in 'training age':

0-6 months – beginner: Someone who has never previously exercised at home or set foot in a gym but has begun to walk or swim, or at least doing some physical activity to get themselves motivated towards their new goal and fitness level.

6-12 months – beginner to intermediate: Someone who has been doing limited activity, such as walking or participating in some group fitness classes, Pilates or yoga.

12-24 months – intermediate: Someone with good or reasonable fitness who is participating in a gym environment with resistance and cardio-type training.

24 months onward – intermediate to advanced: The fitness "guru" who would normally train 4-5 times a week at high intensity or an athlete who loves to be challenged with new or great exercises.

Based on your 'training age', choose a program that is suitable for you, progress only when you are ready, and regress if you find the program is too hard. For example, if you fall into the 0-6 months' category and exercising is easy, you should progress to the next level.

The following terminology is used for completing each exercise:

Sets: The number of times you will complete one particular exercise.

Reps: The number of times you will repeat one movement of exercise.

Tempo: The timing of how fast or how slow you should perform each movement of exercise.

Rest: The amount of time you will take to recover or rest between each set, so that you are ready to repeat another set.

From time to time, I use the word "connect" to remind you to consistently contract your pelvic floor muscles and your deep abdominal muscles, classified as "core muscles". It reminds you to stay connected in order to prevent back pain, and to maintain correct technique.

#D1

CALF RAISES – FREE STANDING – BODY WEIGHT ONLY

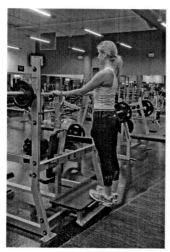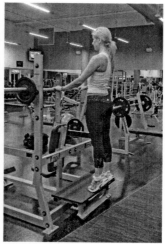

Beginner and Intermediate.

Muscles targeted: Calves and soleus.

Sets: 2 **Reps:** 10-20 **Tempo:** 2:1:3 **Rest:** 60 seconds

Calf stretching and strengthening is very important during your workout as we discussed in the early chapters. Having tight calves will prevent you from squatting effectively. If you are accustomed to wearing high heels, then this exercise should benefit you, as the stretch component under load will balance things out.

1. From a flat-footed position, stand on a step or a platform and gently lower your heels towards the floor, feeling the stretch.

2. Without compromising your posture or bending your knees, lift and come up completely on your toes (the balls of your feet) feeling your calves contract.

3. Tempo is up for 2 counts, hold for 1 count and lower it down slowly for 3 counts. Lowering down slowly will put tension on the muscle while stretching, thus building strength.

4. Start with 2 sets of 10 repetitions and build up to 4 sets of 20 repetitions, with 60 seconds rest between each set.

Tips:

It is a very good idea to do some muscle spasm release (self-myofascial release) on the foam roller for your calves ***before*** you do this exercise.

The next time you are squatting, pay attention to your feet. If you are raising your heels off the floor when you are in a full squat position, this may be due to tight calves. Releasing, stretching and strengthening the calves will benefit you in your daily life, as well as in your training.

#D2

CALF RAISES – LOADED – MACHINE

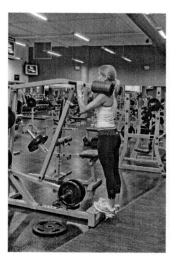 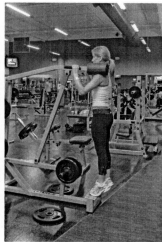

Intermediate and Advanced.

Muscles targeted: Calves and soleus.

Sets: 3 **Reps:** 12-20 **Tempo:** 2:1:3 **Rest:** 60 seconds

1. There are several varieties of calf machines available, so choose one that you feel comfortable using.

2. For the machine in this photo, the padded rollers rest on your shoulders, with your feet positioned in an already stretched position.

3. Stand comfortably and raise your heels, feeling the calves contract. Lower yourself down slowly.

4. For intermediate, begin with light-medium weight and do 12 repetitions. As your calf strength increases, so should the weight you lift.

5. Alternatively, stay with the medium weight and increase the repetitions to 20.

6. Advanced people, 3 sets with 12 repetitions with medium to heavy weight.

7. Rest for 60 seconds between each set.

Tip:

See Tips from "beginner" calf raises (exercise #D1).

#D3

Ball Wall Squat

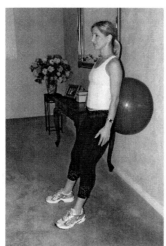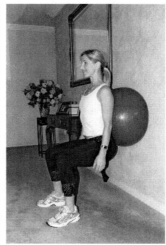

Beginner – a must read for all levels.

Muscles targeted: Legs, gluteus and deep abdominal wall (core).

Sets: 2-4 **Reps:** 10-25 **Tempo:** 3:1:3 **Rest:** 60 seconds

The key here is to breathe through your diaphragm, and it should look like your stomach is expanding. As you breathe out, draw your bellybutton inward, lifting the pelvic floor at the same time – this contracts your core muscles. You need to make sure that it's the lower portion of your stomach that draws inwards. This is the area below the bellybutton.

IT'S ONLY AFTER YOU HAVE DONE THIS THAT YOU ARE READY TO SQUAT. *Notice how effective and fluid your movement will be when you have your pelvic floor muscles contracting with your deep abdominals. If you let go of these, your squats become rushed and messy. I urge you to pay special attention to your squatting. Once you have mastered this, not only* *will you have lovely legs and toned buttocks, but you will have great tummy muscles (and you won't need to do hundreds of sit-ups which incidentally will put unnecessary strain on your neck.)*

1. Position the ball in the small of your back. Place your feet just slightly forward of your hips and slightly wider than hip-width.

2. Breathe and connect all deep abdominal muscles. Squat down slowly for a count of 3, and lower only to a position where you are comfortable. It may be 30 degrees or up to 90 degrees at the knees (as if you are sitting in a chair). Hold that position for 1 count and come up in 3 counts.

3. For an absolute beginner only do 2 sets with 10 repetitions. Tempo is down for 4 counts, hold for 1 and come up in 4 counts.

4. If you have done some ball squatting before, do 15 repetitions and go down for 3 counts, hold for 1 and come up in 3. Go at your own pace, with a minimum of 2 sets of 15 repetitions. Aim for 3 to 4 sets and 15-25 repetitions, focusing on staying connected with your pelvic floor and deep abdominal muscles throughout each set.

Tip:

As you go down in your squat, imagine you are sitting on a chair, and you are tipping the edge of the chair and come back up.

One common observation that I have made with people squatting is that they rush their squats. It's almost pointless doing these if you do not do them properly.

#D4

FRONT BAR SQUAT

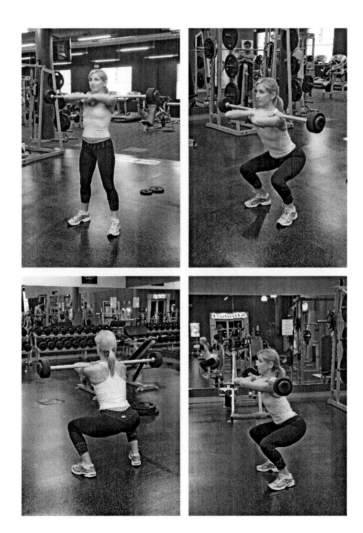

Intermediate and Advanced.

Muscles targeted: Whole body: gluteus, legs, buttocks, upper back and deep abdominal muscles.

Sets: 3-6 **Reps:** 12 **Tempo:** 3:1:2 **Rest:** 60-90 seconds

This exercise is for those of you who have been training for a while and are accustomed to the back squat. I actually prefer to teach my clients the front squat as I can concentrate on technique and train their upper back at the same time while keeping their spine long.

If you still prefer to do the back squat, then move to using a squat rack. Mix it up and have a friend train with you to spot you with the front squat, until you become confident with the technique.

1. Start with a light 10kg bar, until you get used to the positioning on your arms and keeping the core activated and stabilised.

2. Place the bar evenly either side, just in front of the cut at the shoulder and bicep muscles. Cross your arms, placing opposite hand to opposite shoulder. Keep your arms elevated but the shoulders depressed. This will ensure that you are using the scapula muscles (shoulder blade muscles) to stabilise the shoulder and to contract the "weaker" rhomboid muscles (mid back muscles).

3. Before you start to squat down, breathe in and as you breathe out, connect all your deep abdominal muscles.

4. Make sure that your pelvic floor muscles are contracted (not a sharp tight squeeze) it should be a comfortable lift and maintained the whole time you are squatting. (This will ensure that your "multifidus" muscles contract – which is a long muscle that goes from the base of your spine and all the way down to the tailbone. You need this muscle working as it supports your spine - the only time it contracts is when your pelvic floor is contracted.)

5. Squat down for 3 counts, hold for 1 and come up in 2 counts while breathing out through your lips. Push through your glutes to get you that lift.

6. If your heels are lifting off the floor, stop and stretch your calves to lower them back to the floor – this will make your squats much more effective.

7. Time your rest period, as this is also important, as the core muscles need adequate rest to protect your lower back.

Tip:

For the more intermediate to advanced squatter, notice I have suggested 6 sets. I invite you to challenge yourself and get stronger before your pregnancy. Simply add an extra set with some extra weight each time you train legs and you will become stronger.

#D5

SINGLE ARM DEAD ROW/PULL – CABLE

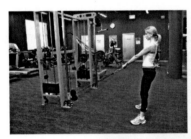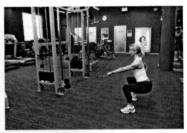

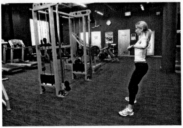

Intermediate.

Muscles targeted: Whole body.

Sets: 3 **Reps:** 12 **Tempo:** 3:1:2 **Rest:** 60 seconds

This is a great exercise as it involves the legs, core and back muscles, all in one movement. This exercise is performed on a cable machine. All cable machines come with various attachments for different exercises or movements. Attach a handle that resembles a horseshoe.

1. Start with your feet **wider** than hip-width apart and the handle in your left hand.

2. Breathe in; as you breathe out, draw your bellybutton in towards your spine and lift your pelvic floor muscles.

3. Hold that as you lower into your squat position for 3 counts.

4. As you come up in 2 counts, breathe out and pull with your left arm until your elbow goes past your ribcage and you feel the squeezing in your back.

5. Keep your shoulder and upper traps (neck/shoulder muscles) relaxed.

6. Do 12 repetitions with each arm and repeat for 3 sets.

7. Essentially, you will get a total of 24 squats out of each set.

Tip:

You can also do this exercise with both arms pulling – however you will need a rope that is used for triceps work.

#D6 & #D7

HIP EXTENSION LEG CURL WITH SWISS BALL

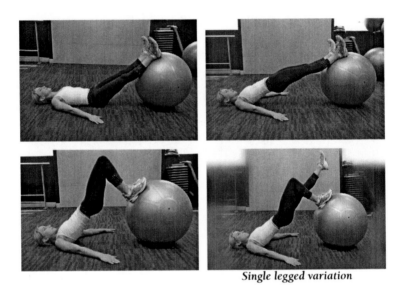

Single legged variation

Beginner and Intermediate.

Muscles targeted: Hamstrings, calves, hips and core.

Sets: 2-4 **Reps:** 12-20 **Tempo:** 2:1:3 **Rest:** 60 seconds

If only all exercise was as easy as lying on the floor and getting it done and out of the way! Well this time it is!

One of my favourite hamstring exercises is the leg curl on the ball. This exercise will help you balance weak muscles as well as create stability and strength in your hips and buttocks.

1. Lie on your back with the ball positioned under your calves and heels. Relax your shoulder and neck with palms down for support.

2. Connect your deep abdominal wall with pelvic floor muscles before you lift. When you are ready, lift your hips up. Stabilise. With your heels, bring the ball close to your buttocks for 2 counts. Hold for 1 count, and go back to full extension in 3 counts.

3. Repeat this sequence in a controlled manner.

4. For absolute beginners, start with 2 sets of 10 repetitions with same tempo and 60 second rest. Build it up to 3 sets.

5. For intermediate do 3 to 4 sets with 20 repetitions.

6. Rest for 60 seconds between each set and stretch the hamstrings if they are tight. There is no need to stretch if you are normally quite flexible.

Tips:

This is a fantastic exercise to do before your squats. I have found that performing leg curls before squats warms up the hamstrings and glutes. By doing this exercise first you will perform better quality squats and possibly less knee pain if that has been an issue.

For advanced people, doing 1-legged single leg curls works really well. These have the same starting position, but lift one leg off the ball and maintain same alignment with hips and body, curl one leg for 12 repetitions and same tempo. Focus on your hamstring and buttocks working. Repeat on the other side and rest for 60 seconds. Attempt 4 sets and you should really feel the hamstrings strengthen. I do not recommend stretching after this exercise.

#D8

LEG PRESS MACHINE

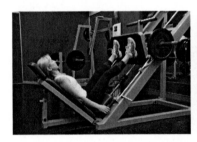 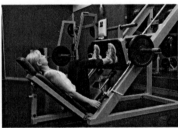

Beginner, Intermediate and Advanced.

Muscles targeted: Front and back of thighs, buttocks, calves and core.

Sets: 2-4 **Reps:** 12-20 **Tempo:** 3:1:2 **Rest:** 60-90 seconds

My preferred option and exercise for the legs and buttocks is a front squat. However, at times, I find the leg press machine quite useful, as women who psychologically can't lift heavy weight in a squat prefer the support of a leg press machine.

There are varieties of machines available, but your seating position is the same.

1. Make sure you are sitting in the middle of the seat and that your legs are equally positioned on the platform.

2. Push your bottom right back in the seat and never lift off the seat during your pushing or lowering of the weight.

3. At this point, please never adjust your sitting while your legs are under load.

4. In the photograph, there is a bar with holes and a pin. This is right in front of your seat, and between your legs. This bar is very useful and you should position the pin in one of the holes half way up, so that if the weight is too heavy and you cannot push the weight back, it acts as a "catch". Ask for assistance in your gym if you are not sure.

5. Sit back on the seat, with legs extended and feet slightly wider than hip-width apart.

6. Breathe in through your deep abdominal wall. Breathe out, and draw your belly button in, contracting your pelvic muscles. Lower the platform in 3 counts until your knees reach at 90 degrees.

7. Breathe out while pushing back up with your bellybutton still contracting your tummy.

8. If you are just starting on the leg press, do 20 repetitions with light weight, and progress on to heavier weight as you go along. Aim to get 12 repetitions with reasonable weight. Rest for 60 seconds.

9. If you do leg presses regularly, increase the weight so that the last 4 repetitions of your 12 are starting to burn. Tempo is always the same. Building strength requires slow coming down for 3 counts and holding it for 1. Get the glutes really fired up and burning on that 1 count and then push the weight back up for 2 counts.

10. Make sure you stay connected with your pelvic floor muscles when you push the platform back up, so that at each repetition you have quality contraction in your core and are protecting your lower back.

11. Depending on the load, you may need rest for 60-120 seconds. If you are lifting heavier weight, then you need a longer rest period.

Tip:

Hips are generally tight on most people. After the leg press, it is a good idea to do a thigh stretch. See exercise #B13 *Hip Flexor with the Swiss Ball.*

#D9

LUNGE ON THE SWISS BALL

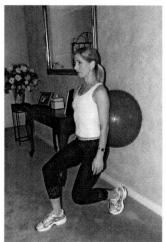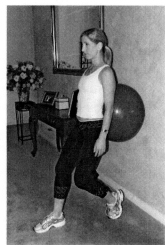

Beginner and Intermediate.

Muscles targeted: Front and back of thighs and core.

Sets: 2-4 **Reps:** 12 **Tempo:** 3:1:2 **Rest:** 60 seconds

This is such a great exercise! Amazing strength takes place when you do single leg lunge or squat. If you love having toned buttocks and back of your legs – this is for you. From stability perspective, it really works on the strength of your hips.

1. Position the ball on the small of your back, so that you feel supported. Take your right leg forward and the left leg back. To allow a correct and effective lunge action, you must lift your left heel off the floor.

2. Stand tall with your ribcage lifted, shoulders in line with hips and take in a breath. As you breathe out, connect the deep abdominal wall with pelvic floor muscles.

3. Lunge down, as if you are trying to sit back in a chair, to a position that feels comfortable. For most of us going down to 90 degrees feels great, however if you have glute, hip or knee instability, lowering yourself down to 45 degrees may be the most you can accomplish.

4. Stay connected with your midsection the whole time you are moving down and up.

5. **Beginner** – do 2 sets of 12 repetitions; **Intermediate** – do 3 sets of 12 repetitions. And for maximum results, back leg is off the floor – do 4 sets of 12 repetitions.

6. Rest for 60 seconds between each set.

Tip:

Ensure that your hips are at an even level and not dropping on either side. For example if your right leg is forward and you are lunging down, make sure your left hip is staying aligned with the right hip. Lower only to the level where both hips are even.

#D10

LUNGE ON TWO BOSU® BALLS

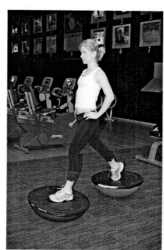 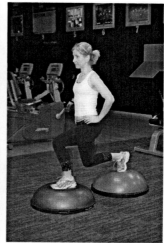

Intermediate.

Muscles targeted: Legs, glutes and core.

Sets: 3 **Reps:** 12 **Tempo:** 3:1:3 **Rest:** 60 seconds

You will notice in some of the pictures that the dome (BOSU®) is facing downwards and in others the dome-side is up. This option enables you to choose the challenge of practising which is more suitable for your fitness level, and also to focus on stability in your core muscles. Try it with the flat section on the floor first, working on stabilising your footing on the unstable BOSU®. You can place the BOSU® near a wall for stability, or if you are training with a friend, use their hand to balance just enough to get you started.

This is fantastic leg work, to add something different to your routine and also challenge your stability, strength and balance.

1. Place one BOSU® at the front, and the other is behind and slightly to the side of the front BOSU®. Stabilise and balance by connecting deep abdominal muscles and pelvic floor.

2. Start with a split stance. Ensure your back foot is loaded on your toes, and your body weight is distributed evenly between the front and back leg.

3. You must have your back foot exactly in the centre of the BOSU®.

4. Once you feel stable on the BOSU®, start to lunge down for a count of 3, hold for 1 count and come up for 3 counts. Perform 12 repetitions.

5. Your focus should be on the balance with the correct lunge technique.

6. When you have completed your 12 repetitions, lower the front BOSU® down with your heel and when you feel safe, take your back foot off the back BOSU®.

7. To do the other side, repeat from step 1 on the opposite side.

Tip:

Getting on and off the BOSU® may prove to be a challenge at the beginning. Align yourself closer to a wall so that you can use some support or a friend's hand. It will take a bit of practice and stability work.

#D11

LUNGE ON THE BOSU® WITH DB BICEP CURLS

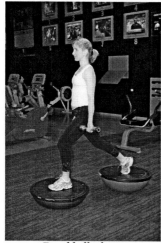 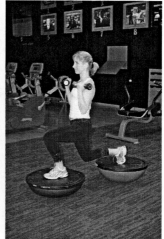

| *Dumbbells down* | *Dumbbells raised* |

Intermediate.

Muscles targeted: Legs, buttocks, core and biceps.

Sets: 3 **Reps:** 12 **Tempo:** 3:1:2 **Rest:** 60-90 seconds

Progression from the basic lunge on the BOSU® can be achieved by adding some dumbbells and performing a variety of arm lines, such as a bicep curl, lateral raise or shoulder press.

These exercises are included so that if you are short on time, you can still do a total body workout in a short session and gain great toning and strengthening benefits.

1. Start with a split stance. Ensure your back foot is loaded on your toes, and your body weight is distributed evenly between front and back leg.

2. You must have your back foot exactly in the middle in the centre of the BOSU®.

3. Use light to medium dumbbells and perform a bicep curl.

4. As you go down for 3 counts, bring the dumbbells up in a curl to the front of your shoulders, with your knuckles facing up. Hold for 1 count, and lower your arms for 2 counts as you come up from your lunge.

5. Concentrate on connecting your pelvic floor and deep abdominal muscles as you return to the starting position.

6. Repeat for 12 repetitions or do as many as you can to begin with and please, always start with a light weight.

7. Repeat on the other side.

8. Rest between each set for 60-90 seconds, as controlling the stability and balance of this movement can be quite challenging.

#D12

LUNGE ON THE BOSU® WITH LATERAL DB RAISE

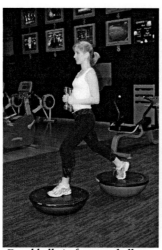

Dumbbells in front and elbows at 90 degrees   *Elbows wide and at 90 degrees*

Intermediate.

Muscles targeted: Legs, glutes, arms and shoulders.

Sets: 3 **Reps:** 12 **Tempo:** 3:1:2 **Rest:** 60-90 seconds

Adding a lateral raise will really make your core muscles work, as your arms are travelling away from your body.

1. Start with a split stance. Ensure your back foot is loaded on your toes, and your body weight is distributed evenly between front and back leg.

2. You must have your back foot right in the middle in the centre of the BOSU®. Use the same posture and stability as in the other BOSU® exercises. Hold your dumbbells as if you are holding 2 full glasses of water.

3. As you go down for 3 counts, carefully take your arms out and as if you are slowly tipping the water out of your glasses for 1 count.

4. Bring the arms down in 2 counts as you come up from your lunge. Refocus every time you go down and up with your lunge, fixing your eyes on a spot on the wall or the floor to help you stabilise.

5. Repeat this for 12 repetitions keeping good form.

6. Turn and do the other side.

7. Rest for 60-90 seconds between each set.

#D13

LUNGE ON BOSU® WITH DB SHOULDER PRESS

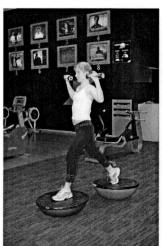 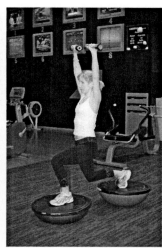

Intermediate.

Muscles targeted: Legs, buttocks, arms and shoulders.

Sets: 3 **Reps:** 12 **Tempo:** 3:1:3 **Rest:** 60-90 seconds

Just when you thought the lateral raises were hard, here is the last one!

1. Start with a split stance. Ensure your back foot is loaded on your toes, and your body weight is distributed evenly between front and back leg. You must have your back foot exactly in the centre of the BOSU®. Use the same posture and stability as for the other BOSU® exercises.

2. Take your arms out to 90 degrees at the elbow and shoulders, so it looks like an L shape at the elbows. As you lunge down for 3 counts your arms come up with a shoulder press. Hold for 1 count, and then return to the starting position for 3 counts.

3. Do as many repetitions as you can – up to 12, while keeping good form. Change legs and do the other side.

4. Rest for 60-90 seconds and repeat.

Tip:

Having the BOSU® with the flat side facing up is easier for balance.

#D14

ROTATIONAL LUNGE WITH A MEDICINE BALL

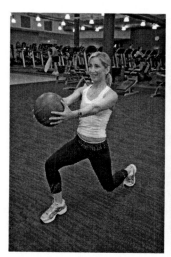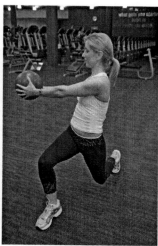

Beginner and Intermediate.

Muscles targeted: Whole body.

Sets: 2 **Reps:** 10-20 **Tempo:** 2:0:2 **Rest:** 30 seconds

Once you have mastered the lunge, either on the ball on the wall or without, your next progression will involve some rotational movement. Remember, you will be twisting with loading and offloading shopping bags or prams from your car.

This is an excellent exercise as it involves the oblique muscles (waist muscles) working with your transverse abdominals.

1. Start with a split stance. Ensure your back foot is loaded on your toes, and your body weight is distributed evenly between the

front and back leg. Connect your pelvic floor and deep abdominal muscles.

2. As you lunge down, rotate to the outside of your front leg keeping your eyes fixed on the medicine ball. Shoulders and arms are relaxed and all movement should be coming from your legs, glutes and midsection.

3. Aim for 10-20 repetitions with good form on each leg, and rest for 30-60 seconds between each set.

4. Lunge down and rotate simultaneously for a count of 2 and come up without resting for a count of 2. Always breathe out as you come up. You may add another set, or if you are feeling strong, use a heavier medicine ball.

Tip:

Your medicine ball can weigh from 1-5kg, depending on your training age and level of strength and fitness. This exercise can also be done with a cable machine at the same tempo. However, be careful to stay in control, as your core muscles should be controlling the pull and release of the weight.

#D15

ROTATIONAL LUNGE AND EXTENSION WITH A MEDICINE BALL

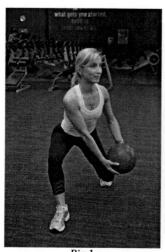 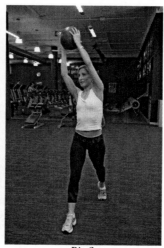

Pic 1   Pic 2

Intermediate.

Muscles targeted: Whole body.

Sets: 2 **Reps:** 10-20 **Tempo:** 2:0:2 **Rest:** 30 seconds

This exercise is the progression of the exercise above, with an extension of the arms up towards the ceiling.

Picking up washing and putting it on the line is the familiar domestic practice with which you can acquaint this exercise.

1. Start with a split stance with feet hip-width apart. Ensure your back foot is loaded on your toes, with your body weight distributed evenly between the front and back leg.

2. Lift your pelvic floor muscles and contract your core muscles before you begin this exercise. As you lunge down, rotate and flex (bend forward and down) on the inside of your front leg. Have your eyes fixed on the medicine ball. Shoulders and arms are relaxed, and all your movement should be from your legs, glutes and midsection (pic 1).

3. Using your glutes, push through your front heel and lift the ball up towards the ceiling with both arms straight, and please **do not lock the elbows**.

4. Extend and feel the lengthening of your torso (pic 2).

5. Repeat on the other side.

6. If you are a beginner with this exercise, then start small with 8 repetitions and going down for 2 counts, without resting come up for 2 counts.

7. If you regularly do lunges, then really focus on the weight of the ball and the extension of your torso, which will give you a fantastic stretch. Try increasing the repetitions to 20, as though you are putting a load of washing on the line.

8. Always breathe out as you come up.

Tip:

Your medicine ball can vary from 1kg-3kg, depending on your training age and level of strength and fitness. Do not have it any heavier, as this may cause your lower back to hyperextend (an excessive arch in the lower back).

#D16

SQUAT WITH A DB EXTENSION OR A SNATCH

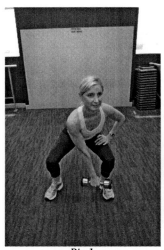 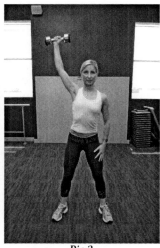

Pic 1   Pic 2

Intermediate and Advanced.

Muscles targeted: Whole body.

Sets: 3 **Reps:** 12 **Tempo:** 2:1:2 **Rest:** 60 seconds

This is another variation of squat with an arm line. Most of us are short on time so we can maximise an exercise and work our upper and lower body at the same time.

1. Stand with your feet **wider** than shoulder-width. Connect your pelvic floor and deep abdominal muscles. Take your right arm across towards your left foot, and go down to a squat position (pic 1). This is your starting position.

2. Do not lose your pelvic floor contraction in the squatted position. This is very important, as it will protect your back during the squat and the lift of the arm. The whole point of this exercise is to tone and strengthen legs and glutes with a variation of upper body involvement. As you come up from the squat, keep your arm in a close position (like playing a guitar) and, when your reach your chest, open the forearm and lift to the ceiling (pic 2).

3. Use a dumbbell that is a comfortable weight for all 12 repetitions. If one arm is weaker, then let the weak arm determine the weight for the other arm.

4. Repeat with the other arm and rest for 60 seconds after you have completed the exercise with both arms.

5. Repeat for 3 sets.

#D17

TORSO CABLE ROTATION

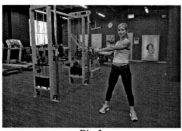

Pic 1	Pic 2

Cable machine is on your right and hold the handle with left hand first

Beginner, Intermediate and Advanced.

Muscles targeted: Torso, shoulders and arms.

Sets: 3 **Reps:** 12 **Tempo:** 2:1:3 **Rest:** 60 seconds

This is a lovely rotational exercise, which involves your whole midsection.

1. It is **very important** that the position of your cable is below your shoulder height. Aim for the handle to be at midsection level.

2. Stand sideways with the cable machine on your right. Hold the handle with your left hand first and your right hand over your left hand. (Vice versa for the other side.)

3. Start with a light weight to begin and progressively increase the weight over time, as your strength increases.

4. Contract your deep abdominal wall and relax your shoulders.

5. Make sure your arms are straight, however ensure that during the movement, your elbows are "soft" (not locked).

6. Pull for a count of 2 to one side while you are contracting your midsection. Hold for 1 count (pic 2) and release for 3 counts.

7. Do 12 repetitions on each side, rest for 60 seconds and repeat the set.

#D18

WOOD CHOP – CABLE MACHINE

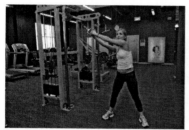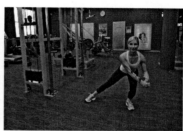

Intermediate and Advanced.

Muscles targeted: Whole body.

Sets: 3 **Reps:** 12 **Tempo:** 2:1:3 **Rest:** 60-90 seconds

Wood chop is one of the most commonly prescribed functional exercises. It targets the whole body with flexion (forward bending) and extension (opposite to forward bending), thus making it applicable to most daily activities.

Here I have used the cable machine and facing sideways with feet wider than hips. If you are just starting with this exercise, you can begin with your feet closer and just perform the wood chop, without shifting and using your legs and glutes.

1. Stand with a tall posture, relax your shoulders and activate your deep abdominal wall and pelvic floor muscles.

2. Hold the handle with your left hand if you are wood chopping to the left side, and your right hand over the left.

3. Start with body weight loaded on the right leg. As you go through your wood chop transfer and squat on the left leg.

4. If you are more of an **intermediate** person, allow your right leg to extend (be straight), and get a lovely inner thigh stretch.

5. If you are just starting with the wood chop, then balance your bodyweight evenly over both legs i.e. normal squat position.

6. Chop for 2 counts, maintaining great posture, and use your mid-section to do all the work with the pull. Hold for 1 count and return to the starting position in a slow and controlled movement for 3 counts.

7. Repeat the other side.

8. Perform 12 repetitions with 3 sets and 60-90 seconds rest between each set.

Caution!

If you have lower back issues, use caution with this exercise. Seek medical advice and if cleared, commence with light weight.

#D19

REVERSE WOOD CHOP – CABLE

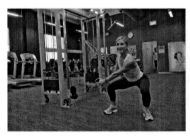 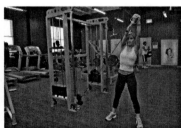

Intermediate and Advanced.

Muscles targeted: Whole body.

Sets: 3 **Reps:** 12 **Tempo:** 2:1:3 **Rest:** 60-90 seconds

Reverse Wood Chop is the opposite of the wood chop exercise. (see exercise #D18)

1. Prepare the cable with the handle at the bottom of the machine. Stand sideways to the cable machine.

2. As your starting position is in the **squat**, you must breathe in and out using your diaphragm and contract your deep abdominal wall and pelvic floor muscles *before* you assume the squat position.

3. Maintain core activation; the emphasis here is using your glutes, legs and core to pull up for 2 counts, hold for 1 and release for 3 counts.

4. Complete 12 repetitions with 3 sets and 60-90 seconds rest between each set.

Tip:

To begin with and to help get your technique right, always start with lighter weight rather than medium, so that your posture is not compromised, and you can focus on the core being switched on for the entire set.

Caution!

The moment you have lost pelvic floor contraction and core activation, the set is finished.

#D20

PRONE COBRA ON SWISS BALL

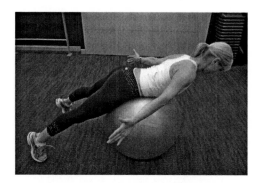

Beginner and Intermediate.

Muscles targeted: Upper, mid and lower back.

Sets: 2 **Reps:** 8-12 **Tempo:** 2:2:2 **Rest:** 30-60 seconds

This is can be for beginners, but it's mostly an intermediate exercise. For the beginner's version, prone cobra can be performed on the floor using the same technique.

This is a great warm up exercise especially for the days when you are concentrating on training your back.

1. Lie on your tummy on the ball and relax over the Swiss ball as if you are hugging it.

2. Breathe in and as you breathe out, draw your bellybutton in and away from the ball, contracting your pelvic floor muscles at the same time (you may squeeze your glutes also).

3. Lift both arms up and rotate outwards with thumbs pointing backwards (towards the ceiling).

4. Do not hyperextend your neck; make sure you are facing the floor.

5. Push your shoulder blades down towards the hips. Hold for 2 counts.

6. Release and repeat for 8 to 12 repetitions in total.

7. Rest for 60 seconds between each set.

#D21

Single Arm Cable Pull

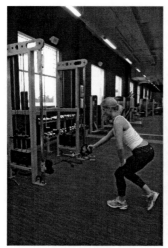 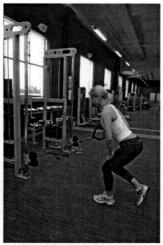

Left leg forward, handle in right hand   *Draw the handle toward your body*

Beginner, Intermediate and Advanced.

Muscles targeted: Whole body.

Sets: 3 **Reps:** 12 **Tempo:** 2:1:3 **Rest:** 60 seconds

1. Set the cable pulley to a low position.

2. Starting position is with a split stance. Your left leg is forward and your right leg is back, making sure you are on your toes on your right foot; this will give you greater rotation.

3. Your opposite hand (right) is holding the handle of the cable machine.

4. Lengthen and flex your body at 45 degrees, with the curvature in your lower back and shoulders relaxed.

5. Breathe in; as you breathe out, draw your bellybutton in towards your spine as you contract your pelvic floor.

6. Maintain this contraction throughout the set.

7. Pull the cable for 2 counts, hold contraction in the shoulder blade for 1 count and release for 3 counts.

8. Complete 12 repetitions, with 3 sets with a 60-second rest between each set.

#D22

SEATED ROW – CABLE, BALL OR MACHINE

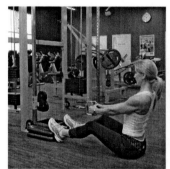

Handle in front of your knees

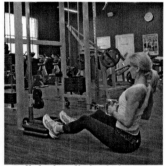

Pull the handle back, keeping the contraction in your middle back and your chest elevated

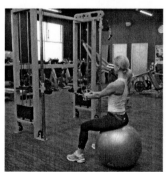

Swiss ball version

Beginner, Intermediate and Advanced.

Muscles targeted: Back (rhomboids) and biceps.

Sets: 3 **Reps:** 12 **Tempo:** 2:1:3 **Rest:** 60 seconds

If you choose to breastfeed, you will need to strengthen this area, as holding your baby repeatedly in a feeding position can otherwise potentially lead to a rounded back and poor posture.

I have used the cable machine, however there are some very good seated-rowing machines available which can work equally as well.

1. Sit on the floor or machine with an upright posture, knees bent and holding the handle just in front of your knees.

2. Activate your deep abdominal wall and contract your pelvic floor muscles.

3. Breathe in; as you breathe out, pull for 2 counts and hold for 1 count.

4. Maintain contraction in the middle of your back while your chest is in an elevated position. Release slowly for 3 counts.

5. **For beginners**, the Swiss ball is a great way to start – perform 15 repetitions with a lighter weight. **For the intermediate** level, go slightly heavier than you are accustomed to.

6. Rest for 60 seconds between each set.

Tips:

Keep your head aligned with the rest of your spine and avoid a forward head posture during movement.

If you find yourself sliding forward, use a riser or platform to steady your feet as shown.

#D23

SEATED HIGH ROW – MACHINE

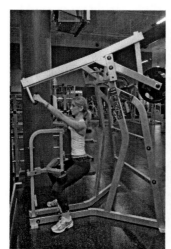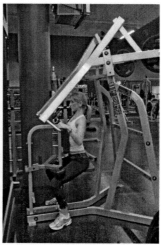

Beginner, Intermediate and Advanced.

Muscles targeted: Back and biceps.

Sets: 3 **Reps:** 12 **Tempo:** 2:1:3 **Rest:** 60 seconds

There are a wide variety of back machines available, from the well-known Lateral Pull-down, to many types of adjustable cable machines.

The high row machine in the picture was chosen because it is more user-friendly for those with shoulder issues. The arms don't go out as with the Lat Pull-down machine, thus making it easier on the shoulders.

1. Adjust the seat so that you are not squashed behind it, and you are sitting tall but comfortably.

2. Align your neck with your spine. Keep your tongue on the roof of your mouth and tuck in your chin comfortably. (This ensures you do not strain the back of your neck.)

3. Relax your shoulders and with your shoulder blades down and slightly drawn towards your spine).

4. Activate your core muscles and then pull evenly with both arms for 2 counts, contracting the back. Hold for 1 count and release for 3 counts.

5. Repeat for 12 repetitions and 3 sets.

6. If you are a **beginner**, you may wish to begin with a lighter weight and complete 20 repetitions.

7. For the **intermediate** level, complete 12 repetitions, as you should focus on heavier weight for strength.

8. Rest for 60 seconds between each set.

#D24

PRONE JACK KNIFE – TUMMY TUCK

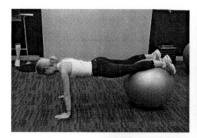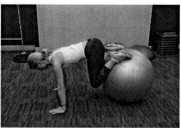

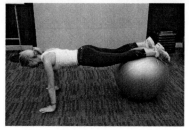

Intermediate.

Muscles targeted: Inner and outer abdominal wall.

Sets: 2-4 **Reps:** 12 **Tempo:** 2:1:3 **Rest:** 60-90 seconds

I love to call this exercise the "Tummy Tuck"! Because the lower abdominals tend to hang around and the loose skin just sits there, this is an area many post-pregnant women complain about. So it's important that you really work this exercise.

The Prone Jack Knife was introduced to me some 15 years ago, and I give this abdominal exercise to almost all of my clients.

I must stress that beginners should not do this straight away. When I start a client with this exercise, I am careful to spot them very well, so that they don't fall off or sink in the middle.

1. Start by rolling yourself on the ball until your shins are well supported on top of the ball.

2. Stabilise your upper body with your arms and through your chest and shoulder blades, avoiding the rounded back look.

3. Maintain a plank or bridge-like position and contract your core muscles by lifting your bellybutton up away from the floor.

4. As you tighten the lower abdominals, you will feel your tummy tense up, just by being in that position.

5. Bring your knees towards your chest, as if you are doing a tummy tuck in a count of 2.

6. Hold that position for 1 count, and as you roll back for a count of 3, really focus on the tension of your abdominal area below your bellybutton.

7. When your legs go back, complete the return with perfectly straight legs, almost to a locked-knee position. When you have done this, you will feel the tension in the abdomen again.

8. For intermediate and advanced levels, go for the full 4 sets of 12 repetitions. If you are doing the 4 sets, make sure you take adequate rest time of 90 seconds.

#D25

OBLIQUE TWIST WITH FEET ON THE SWISS BALL

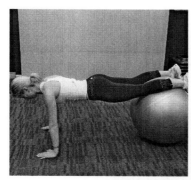
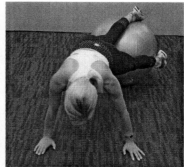

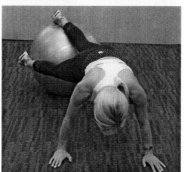

Intermediate and Advanced.

Muscles targeted: Deep abdominal muscles, pelvic floor, obliques-front and back, chest and arms.

Sets: 2-4 **Reps:** 8-16 **Tempo:** 3:1:3 **Rest:** 90-120 seconds

1. Roll forward over the Swiss ball until your shins are resting over the ball.

2. Use the same breathing pattern as Prone Jack Knife (tummy tuck, exercise #D24).

3. Ensure your hips do not drop towards the floor.

4. Keep your body long and stable through your midsection.

5. Connect your core muscles, and then grip the ball with both feet and roll to one side, come back up to the middle, roll to the other side, all in controlled movement for 3 counts.

6. Start with 8 repetitions in total, and build on to 16 repetitions keeping good form for 3 sets. Rest for 90-120 seconds between each set, as you may require longer recovery time.

7. As you become stronger you can change the tempo to 2:1:2 and do more repetitions, ensuring your technique is safe and maintained throughout every movement. Avoid sinking your hips down and putting unnecessary pressure on your lower back.

Tip:

Some clients have been able to manage as many as 30 repetitions total with 4 sets.

#D26

Oblique Twist With Tuck – Lower Body

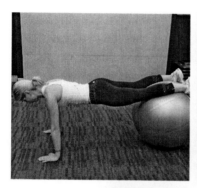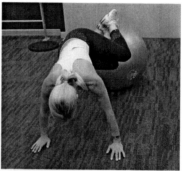

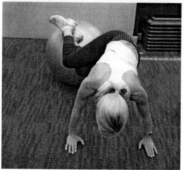

Intermediate and Advanced.

Muscles targeted: Deep abdominal wall, pelvic floor, obliques-front and back, chest and arms.

Sets: 2-4 **Reps:** 8-16 **Tempo:** 2:1:2 **Rest:** 90-120 seconds

This is an intermediate to advanced abdominal exercise. Please be sure you are strong in your mid-section before attempting this.

1. Roll forward over the ball, until your shins are resting over the top of the ball.

2. Feet apart will provide better stability and an easier option, while closer footing will add a challenge to the abdominals.

3. Use the same breathing pattern as the Prone Jack Knife (tummy tuck, exercise #D24).

4. As you tuck your knees in, start twisting to one side for a count of 2, hold that position for 1 count, then return to your starting position for a count of 2.

5. Throughout your twisting, make sure you keep the same hip alignment, slightly elevated and not dropping down to the floor.

6. Complete 8-16 repetitions in total, for 2-4 sets with 90-120 seconds rest between sets. Go at your own pace, and only do what your strength will allow you to do while maintaining good form. Start small and build up.

7. When you finish your set, don't drop to your knees, rather roll yourself backwards over the ball.

Tip:

Be sure to lengthen your body and extend your legs on each return to the starting position.

#D27

OBLIQUE – SIDE CRUNCH ON THE SWISS BALL

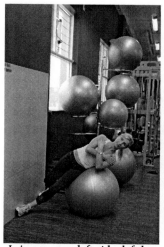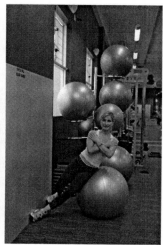

Lying on your left side, left leg forward

Beginner, Intermediate and Advanced.

Muscles targeted: Deep abdominal wall, pelvic floor, obliques-front and back.

Sets: 2-4 **Reps:** 10-20 **Tempo:** 2:1:3 **Rest:** 60-90 seconds

Do you want to get rid of your love handles before you fall pregnant, and after pregnancy? This one simple, effective and safe exercise will do that. It will also give you those lovely lines on your tummy looking like an athlete.

1. Stand sideways to the wall and with your hand holding on the ball. Go into a lunge position with your legs, so that the leg that is closer to the ball goes to the front, and the other leg is back.

2. Lean on to the ball with your hip and position yourself so that you are directly sideways on your hip. Place your feet in a flat position on the wall, not on the floor. This will ensure proper alignment of your ankle and body.

3. Lower yourself sideways to a comfortable position until you feel tension in your waist and abdominal area.

4. For **beginners**, this is the safe position for you to perform 10 repetitions. Side bend (down towards the floor) for count of 3, hold it for 1 count and squeeze your obliques as you come up for 2 counts.

5. For **intermediate levels**, start by performing the same movement as the beginners, but do 20 repetitions on each side, before you progress to holding a medicine ball, dumbbell or a weight plate close to your chest and performing fewer repetitions.

6. Select a medicine ball that is of medium weight, enough to perform 12 repetitions on each side, before moving on to a heavier ball or weight.

7. For **advanced level,** hold a weighted plate or medicine ball away from your chest with arms extended out, or progressively move it up above your head. Again, use caution with the heavy weight, as this is quite a challenging abdominal exercise.

8. Use the same tempo for intermediate and advanced, however your rest period will be longer – up to 120 seconds.

9. Always begin with 2 sets and progressively build up to your level of strength and repetitions.

Tip:

Having your knees bent, particularly the front, will work your waist most effectively and prevent you from cheating. If your front leg is straight, you will be pushing into that leg instead of using the strength of your obliques (waist).

Caution!

Make sure that you're not experiencing lower back stiffness, as this can have an effect on you performing this exercise causing strain on your back instead of strengthening it.

#D28

Alternative Upper Abdominal Exercise

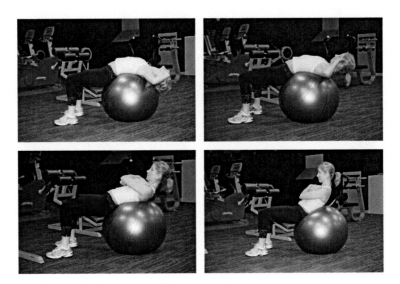

Muscles targeted: Rectus abdominals.

Sets: 2-4 **Reps:** 10-20 **Tempo:** 2:1:3 **Rest:** 60 seconds

How many times have you tried to perform a crunch and it hurts your neck before you start to feel your abdominals? According to experts in rehabilitation, engaging your neck (cervical spine) before your crunch is recommended, as this will also strengthen your neck. Follow the instructions carefully, particularly point 5.

1. Lie on the Swiss ball with your lower back wrapped around the ball.

2. Ensure your head is on the ball and resting comfortably.

3. Place your tongue at the roof of your mouth.

4. Draw your deep abdominal wall in.

5. Do not lift your head off the ball; rather, roll up one vertebra at a time until your chin almost touches your collar bone.

6. It is only now you can perform the crunch with good form.

7. The number of repetitions will vary from person to person. You may only manage 8 at first, but you can progress from there.

8. As soon as you feel any soreness in your neck, stop the crunch, even though you may not feel your abdominals burning.

Tip:

You can also have your hands across the chest, while still curling and lifting the head with the same technique.

#D29

ABDOMINAL PIKE ON SWISS BALL

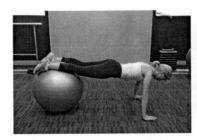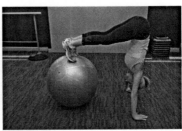

Advanced and Athlete.

Muscles targeted: Deep abdominal wall, pelvic floor muscles, chest, shoulders arms and back.

Sets: 3 Reps: 12 Tempo: 1:2:3 Rest: 90 seconds

This is an advanced exercise and should only be attempted if you have been training with the Swiss ball for a considerable time or if you are an athlete or working with a trainer.

1. Connect your pelvic floor and your deep abdominal muscles before you begin any movement.

2. With both feet, use your toes get a good grip on the Swiss ball and roll it towards your chest.

3. Explosively lift your lower body up towards the ceiling for 1 count. Hold that position for 2 counts, while your head is in neutral position, facing the ball.

4. Contract your abdominal wall, and lower yourself down for 3 counts.

Tips:

Maintain your hip height at the ball level. Do not drop down as you come back down from the pike position.

It is very important to lower yourself down slowly, as the stretching component of the exercise gives strength and stability, calling on all the abdominal muscles.

#D30

PUSH–UP – FLOOR VERSION

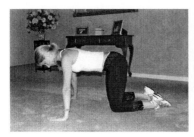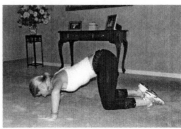

Beginner.

Muscles targeted: Chest and core.

Sets: 2 **Reps:** 10 **Tempo:** 3:1:2 **Rest:** 30-60 seconds

1. Start from a 4-point kneeling position. Ensure that your hands are directly in line with your shoulders and slightly on the outside of your shoulders. Your knees are directly under your hips and hip-width apart.

2. Relax your shoulders and imagine your shoulder blades drawn towards your hips.

3. Breathe in through your stomach (let your tummy expand towards the floor). As you breathe out, use the lower part of your tummy (deep abdominal muscles) to lift your tummy up (belly button towards the spine) and lift your pelvic floor muscles.

4. Do not flatten your lower back out. Maintain the natural curvature by sticking your glutes out.

5. Lower your chest to the floor in 3 counts, hold for 1 count, and come up in 3 counts. Do as many as your midsection and chest will allow.

6. You may start with 5 or 10 repetitions and build it up to the next level. Rest for 30-60 seconds and repeat. As you become stronger, add more repetitions or another set.

Tips:

Learn to do your push-ups correctly using the floor version before you progress.

Do not shrug your shoulders as you go down towards the floor.

#D31

PUSH–UP – WALL VERSION

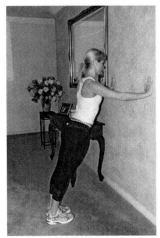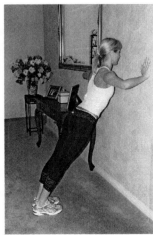

Beginner.

Muscles targeted: Chest, triceps (back of arms) and core.

Sets: 3 **Reps:** 10 **Tempo:** 3:1:2 **Rest:** 60 seconds

1. Stand away from the wall until your arms are reaching the wall and are comfortable at shoulder height.

2. Place your palms on the wall ensuring you do not lock your elbows.

3. Stand tall; let your chest go towards the wall in 3 counts, hold for 1 count and push away from the wall in 2 counts.

4. Ensure you connect your pelvic floor and deep abdominal muscles in. Your elbows are out at 90 degrees and slightly below shoulder height.

5. Complete 10 repetitions for 3 sets. Rest for 60 seconds between each set.

#D32

PUSH–UPS ON THE WALL WITH SWISS BALL

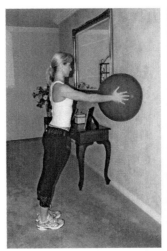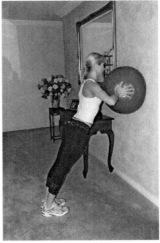

Beginner.

Muscles targeted: Chest, triceps (back of arms) and core.

Sets: 2 **Reps:** 10-15 **Tempo:** 3:1:2 **Rest:** 60 seconds

There are some women who are not able to put pressure on their hands to do push-ups. This is a great alternative, as you can place your hands on the outside of the ball and still manage to do this exercise.

1. Stand away from the wall and ball until your arms are stretched out. Place your hands on either side of the ball. Ensure you connect your pelvic floor and deep abdominal muscles in before you begin your push-up.

2. Your shoulder, elbows and hands should be just below the shoulder height, with elbows slightly bent. Bring your chest towards the ball for a count of 3, hold for 1 count and push away from the ball for a count of 2.

3. Ensure your hips are not the primary move. Use your chest to go towards the ball (not your hips) and keep your hips aligned with your shoulders.

4. Do 2 sets of 10 repetitions, progressing to 15 as you become stronger.

#D33

PUSH–UP – KNEES VERSION

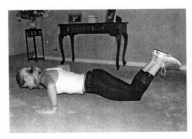 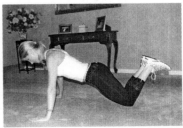

Intermediate.

Muscles targeted: Chest, triceps and core.

Sets: 3 **Reps:** 15 **Tempo:** 3:1:2 **Rest:** 60 seconds

The next progression is the push-up floor version on your knees. Even though this is a chest exercise, I want to stress its importance for the tummy. Too many women compromise their lower back in the gym and during outdoor training. If your hips go down to the floor first, rather than the chest, regress to the beginners' push-up.

1. Your chest and hips should be evenly aligned. In other words, your spine should be in a neutral position from the neck all the way down to your tailbone.

2. Connect your pelvic floor and deep abdominal muscles. Lower yourself down for 3 counts, hold for 1 count and come up in 2, ensuring you are breathing out as you come up.

Tip:

If you have a flat lower back, tilt your pelvis forward to create curvature in your lower back – you will feel the abdominals work more effectively.

Caution!

If your hips come up secondary to your chest on the way up, regress to the beginners' push-up.

#D34

PUSH–UP – FLOOR VERSION

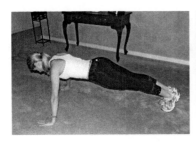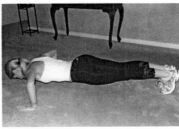

Intermediate and Advanced.

Muscles targeted: Chest, triceps and core.

Sets: 3 Reps: 12 Tempo: 2:1:2 **Rest:** 60 seconds

1. Position yourself on all fours. Place your arms well outside the chest, and your elbows slightly lower than shoulder level.

2. Connect your pelvic floor and deep abdominal muscles before you commence the push-up.

3. Lower yourself down for 2 counts, hold for 1 and, while breathing out, come up in 2.

4. Repeat for 12 repetitions with 60-second rest between each set.

5. If you are feeling strong and want to do more, increase your repetitions to 15 or even 20. However, pay attention to the tempo because 2:1:2 is quite fast; be careful not to not compromise your technique and strength for higher repetitions. As you lower your chest down with slow tempo, your chest is being stretched under tension, therefore it builds strength.

6. The aim is to lower your chest as low as possible. If you are only managing half way down, this exercise is too advanced for you and you should regress to doing push-ups from your knees. Ensure your neck is not compromised by allowing your head to drop down or lift up during the entire push-up time. This occurs all the time in gyms – people are injuring their necks with an incorrect push-up movement.

Tip:

If you want a challenge for your 10 repetitions, then take one foot (barely) off the floor for 5 repetitions and swap over to the other leg for another 5 repetitions. This will give you greater abdominal strength while performing the push-up.

#D35

PUSH–UP ON THE SWISS BALL

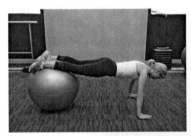 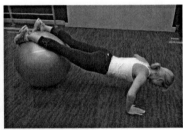

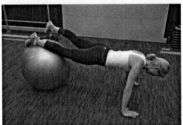

Left leg away from the ball

Intermediate and Advanced.

Muscles targeted: Chest, triceps and core and upper body.

Sets: 3 Reps: 12 Tempo: 3:1:2 **Rest:** 60-90 seconds

This push-up has two versions. The first is with both feet and legs on the Swiss ball. The second is more challenging by taking one leg off the ball, therefore challenging the whole body to perform a full push-up.

1. Roll forward on the Swiss ball until your shins and toes are supported on the top.

2. Place your arms/hands out and well away from the chest.

3. Connect your pelvic floor and deep abdominal muscles in, and maintain full alignment in the torso.

4. Lower yourself down for 3 counts, hold for 1. Come up and breathe out for 2 counts.

5. Complete 6 push-ups with one leg/foot away from the ball, and gently swap over to the other leg for 6 repetitions maintaining good form.

6. If you are able to do 12 repetitions with one leg off and swapping on to the other leg, then go ahead.

7. Complete 3 sets with 60-90 seconds rest between each set.

Caution!

Do not progress to the leg off the ball until you are strong enough to maintain good form. Your lower back should not sway down towards the floor as you lower your chest.

#D36

DB CHEST PRESS ON BENCH

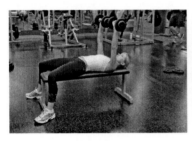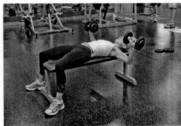

Beginner, Intermediate and Advanced.

Muscles targeted: Chest and triceps.

Sets: 2-4 **Reps:** 12-20 **Tempo:** 3:1:2 **Rest:** 60-90 seconds

If stability is an issue and you are not able to use the Swiss ball yet, your next best option would be to use the bench. This will allow you to get good technique with the dumbbells and as you work through your stability exercises, you can then progress to the ball.

1. Lie on the bench with your head supported on the bench.

2. Take the dumbbells up and over your chest (not your face). Leave a small gap between your lower back and the bench.

3. Even though you are supported on the bench, you still need to connect your pelvic floor and deep abdominal wall, without flattening your back to the bench.

4. Lower the dumbbells down for 3 counts, until your elbows are bent at almost 90 degrees.

5. **Beginners** start with 2 sets of 12 repetitions and light weights, progressing later to medium weight and more sets.

6. **Intermediate to advanced**, choose heavier weight and aim for 3 good sets of 12 repetitions. If you choose to do 4 sets, make sure you have adequate rest between each set.

Caution!

Do not lower your elbows below 90 degrees as your shoulder joint will be compromised. Avoid the risk of injury.

#D37

CHEST PRESS ON A MACHINE

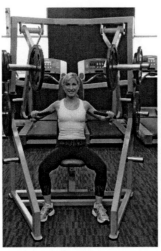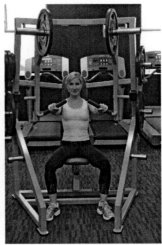

Beginner, Intermediate and Advanced.

Muscles targeted: Chest and triceps.

Sets: 3 **Reps:** 12-20 **Tempo:** 2:1:3 **Rest:** 60 seconds

When using a machine for the chest, be sure you are seated correctly. Most machines have a pin-loaded seat that will allow you to adjust the height. If unsure, ask for assistance from staff at the gym.

1. Place your hands on the handles at a level that will be at the same height or slightly lower than your chest.

2. Use a light weight to begin with until you are comfortable and strong with this machine.

3. Extend both arms out, drop your shoulders down and sit up-right. Bring the arms back, until your elbows are bent at 90 degrees. Use your chest predominantly to do the pushing and releasing, not your arms.

4. For a **beginner**, perform 20 repetitions with a very light weight, pushing for a count of 2, holding for 1 count and releasing for 3 counts.

5. For **intermediate**, perform 15 repetitions using medium weight at the same tempo.

6. For **advanced**, perform 12 repetitions with heavier weight at the same tempo.

#D38

DB CHEST PRESS ON SWISS BALL

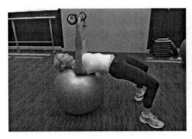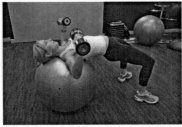

Intermediate and Advanced.

Muscles targeted: Chest, triceps, gluteus, hamstrings and core.

Sets: 3 **Reps:** 12-20 **Tempo:** 3:1:2 **Rest:** 60 seconds

1. Lie on the Swiss ball supporting your shoulders and head. Hold the dumbbells directly over your chest.

2. Line up your hips and glutes with the rest of your body, (or you can have them slightly lower).

3. Place your feet *wider* than hip-width apart, bending your knees at a 90-degree angle.

4. Lower the dumbbells to the side for a count of 3, until your elbows reach 90 degrees (the dumbbell should be directly above your elbow) and hold that position for a count of 1. Push the dumbbells up for 2 counts.

5. Perform 3 sets of 12-20 repetitions with 60-second rest between each set.

#D39

DB CHEST FLYES ON SWISS BALL

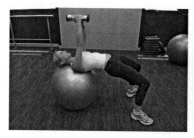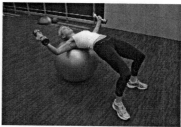

Intermediate.

Muscles targeted: Chest, triceps, gluteus, hamstrings and core.

Sets: 3 **Reps:** 12-20 **Tempo:** 3:1:2 **Rest:** 60 seconds

1. Connect with your core muscles, as for the *DB Chest Press* (exercise #D38).

2. Lie on the ball with arms extended directly above your chest. Hold the dumbbells together.

3. Slowly open your arms for a count of 3, until you feel a stretch in your chest. Do not go below shoulder height. Hold for 1 count and close for a count of 2.

4. Breathe in as you are opening, and breathe out as you close. Maintain your chest in an elevated position.

5. Perform 12 repetitions with medium weight. If you like the feeling of the stretch in your chest and it benefits your posture, you may continue for up to 20 repetitions.

6. Perform total of 3 sets with 60 seconds rest between each set.

#D40

STANDING DB BICEP CURLS

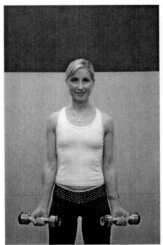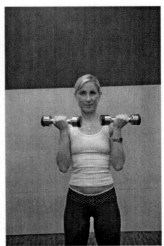

Beginner, Intermediate and Advanced.

Muscles targeted: Biceps and core.

Sets: 2-3 **Reps:** 12-20 **Tempo:** 2:1:3 **Rest:** 60 seconds

You will find that most of the back exercises that I have suggested here involve some pulling movement; hence, they will involve the bicep muscle. Therefore, you may not need to do much isolation work on your biceps.

1. Stand with tall posture, feet hip-width apart and soft at the knees.

2. Arms are down and in front of your thighs.

3. Breathe in and breathe out connecting your pelvic floor and deep abdominal muscles. Relax your shoulders and neck.

4. Curl the arms up with knuckles facing up for 2 counts. Hold for 1 count and lower arms for 3 counts.

5. Continue for total of 12-20 repetitions keeping good form. Start with light dumbbells and increase the weight as you progress with your strength.

6. Complete 3 sets with 60 seconds rest between each set.

Tip:

I have 2-3 sets in the program, however if you would like to get that toned look for your biceps, go for medium weight and do as many as 20 repetitions.

#D41

BICEP CURL – SEATED ON SWISS BALL

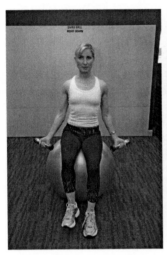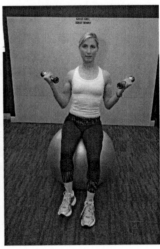

All Fitness Levels.

Muscles targeted: Deep abdominals, pelvic floor, obliques and gluteus medius.

Sets: 3 **Reps:** 12 each side **Tempo:** 2:1:3 **Rest:** 60 seconds

1. Before you attempt bicep curls on the Swiss ball, practice the leg lift for 5-10 seconds without involving the arms.

2. Seated on the ball, connect your pelvic floor and deep abdominal muscles. Visualise your pelvic floor muscles being lifted up and away from the ball.

3. Lift one foot up off the floor and hold.

4. Curl the arms up with knuckles facing up for 2 counts. Hold for 1 count and lower arms for 3 counts. Repeat for 12 reps and lower the leg. Repeat this on each leg.

5. Try not to involve your hip muscles, as this will then defeat the purpose of the exercise. It is not a hip strengthening exercise (hip-flexor exercise), but core stability exercise.

Tips:

Bicep Curls on the ball can be performed with both feet on the floor for a beginner, and for the intermediate and advanced, lift one leg off the floor while performing 12 bicep curls – swap footing and repeat 12 more bicep curls.

Hold the dumbbells comfortably without squeezing them, as squeezing them elevates blood pressure.

#D42

DB LATERAL RAISE–SIDE LIFT

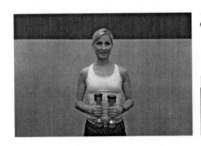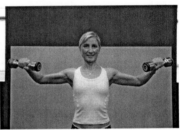

Beginner, Intermediate and Advanced.

Muscles targeted: Shoulders and core.

Sets: 3 **Reps:** 12-20 **Tempo:** 2:1:3 **Rest:** 60 seconds

1. Stand with feet shoulder-width apart and soft at the knees.

2. Hold the dumbbells at bellybutton level as if you have 2 glasses of water in your hands.

3. Relax your shoulders and lift your chest up.

4. Breathe in; as you breathe out, connect your pelvic floor and deep abdominal muscles in.

5. Lift both arms up and out in 2 counts, so that your wrists, elbows and shoulders are at 90 degrees. Hold for 1 count and lower in 3 counts.

6. Maintain neutral neck alignment (do not poke your head forward).

7. Repeat for 12-20 repetitions and 3 sets. Rest for 60 seconds between each set.

#D43

DB Tricep Extension on Swiss Ball – Tricep Kickbacks

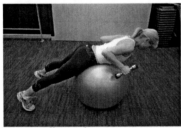 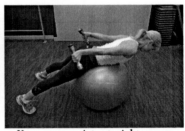

Elbows close to waist   *Keep your wrists straight as you come to full extension with the arms*

Intermediate.

Muscles targeted: Triceps and back.

Sets: 3 **Reps:** 12-20 **Tempo:** 2:1:3 **Rest:** 60 seconds

Prior to attempting this exercise, make sure that your back and deep abdominal wall is strong enough as the lying position on the ball will activate the mid and lower back muscles.

1. Position yourself on the Swiss ball so that you are lying on your tummy and hips. Feet are wide and both arms bent at the elbows holding the dumbbells directly under the shoulders.

2. Keep your head aligned with the rest of the spine and relax your shoulder and upper back muscles. Connect your pelvic floor muscles and your deep abdominal muscles.

3. Extend both arms for 2 counts until you feel the back of your arms contracting. Hold for 1 count and release in 3 counts.

4. Repeat for 12-20 repetitions and 3 sets. Rest for 60 seconds between each set.

Tip:

For advanced, there are better options for working the triceps than lying on the ball. Choose one of the following exercises according to your environment.

#D44

TRICEP DIPS ON BENCH

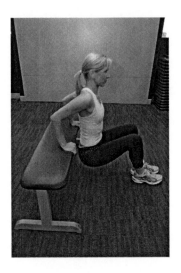

All Fitness Levels.

Muscles targeted: Triceps.

Sets: 3 **Reps:** 12-20 **Tempo:** 3:1:2 **Rest:** 60 seconds

1. Supported on both arms and away from the bench, connect your pelvic floor and deep abdominal muscles.

2. Lift your chest. Place your feet forward enough so that your knees are bent at 90 degrees.

3. Lower your body for a count of 3, staying fairly close to the bench. Hold for 1 count, and return or a count of 2. Ensure your elbows are turned towards the back, and not the side.

4. Perform 12-20 repetitions and 3 sets, with 60 seconds rest between sets.

5. The aim is to go as low as you can, without compromising your shoulders or back. Stay close to the bench with your buttocks.

Tips:

As you become stronger, you can place a weight plate on your lap and use the same tempo – this will add resistance.

Another way to make it more challenging is to take one leg off the floor for 10 repetitions, and swap to the other leg for another 10 repetitions.

Caution!

Do not allow your buttocks to move away from the bench as this will put pressure on your shoulder joint. *Stop immediately* if you feel pressure in your shoulder.

#D45

Tricep Pushdown with a Rope – Cable Machine

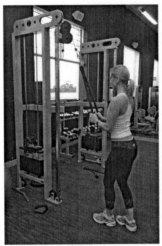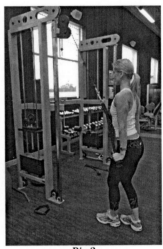

| Pic 1 | Pic 2 |

Beginner, Intermediate and Advanced.

Muscles targeted: Triceps and core.

Sets: 3 **Reps:** 12-20 **Tempo:** 2:1:3 **Rest:** 60 seconds

This is a great isolation exercise for the back of the arms (triceps).

1. This exercise may be performed with a split stance (pic 1 & 2) or with the feet together.

2. Hold the rope at chest level, pull your elbows towards your waist, and contract your core muscles.

3. Lean forward about 20 degrees and with both hands push down for 2 counts, hold for 1 count, and release for 3 counts. You want to feel the back of the arms (triceps) contract. Keep that contraction while you are releasing the rope to the starting position.

4. Make sure that you are not swinging your body forward as you are pushing down.

5. **For beginners**, complete 3 sets of 20 repetitions with light weight.

6. **For intermediate** complete 12 repetitions with medium weight.

7. **For advanced** complete 12 repetitions with medium to heavy weight.

8. Rest for 60 seconds between each set.

Tip:

You can swap the rope for a bar to perform the same exercise. The more you push down and backwards with the rope, the better contraction or activation is achieved in the triceps.

#D46

OVERHEAD TRICEP EXTENSION WITH ROPE ON CABLE MACHINE

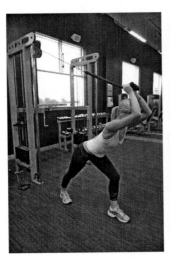 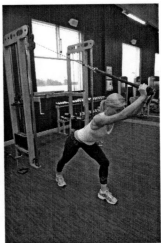

Intermediate and Advanced.

Muscles targeted: Triceps and abdominals.

Sets: 3 **Reps:** 12 **Tempo:** 2:1:3 **Rest:** 60 seconds

This exercise may look like the typical bodybuilder exercise, but it has many more benefits than just the tricep extension. It also opens the chest and torso, while stretching the abdominals.

1. Starting position is a split stance, leaning forward to 45 degrees. Arms up and overhead, holding the rope just above your head.

2. Breathe in and as you breathe out, connect your pelvic floor and deep abdominal muscles. Your posture should be lengthened,

and you should feel your abdominals working. Your spine is in a neutral position with curvature in the lower back.

3. Extend both arms forward in 2 counts, hold for 1 count and return for 3 counts. Breathe out on exertion (pushing).

4. Rest for 60 seconds between each set.

5. Make sure you select the correct weight for your level.

CARDIO STEP UP #DC1

CARDIO STEP UP ON THE STEP #1

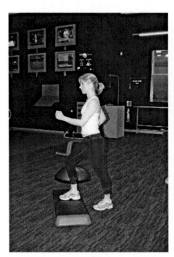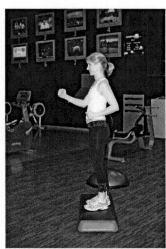

Beginner, Intermediate and Advanced.

Muscles targeted: Whole body.

Sets: minimum 3 **Reps:** 10 each leg
Tempo: medium to fast **Rest:** Nil

At some point in your training, you need to mix some cardio into your weights program. It adds variety and it will keep you motivated. Your heart rate will be up for the entire session, instead of doing cardio before or after weights.

1. Step up for 10 repetitions on each leg. Start with using the platform only. If you are an **intermediate level**, add in the two blocks on each side of step so it is elevated, increasing intensity.

2. With each step, be sure that your whole foot is placed in the middle of the step, and that none of your heel is hanging over the edge, avoiding sore calves.

3. Move your arms in a running action. It will motivate you to see yourself moving at such pace. Tempo should be quite fast with good control so that you don't fall off the step.

Tip:

There are many ways of incorporating the stepping into your weights program. See the program charts for my recommendations.

CARDIO STEP UP #DC2

CARDIO STEP UP #2 – ON BOSU® BALL (DOME)

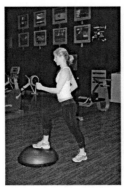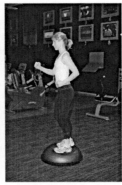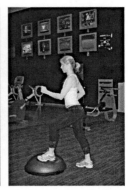

Intermediate and Advanced.

Muscles targeted: Whole body.

Sets: minimum 3 **Reps:** 10 each leg
Tempo: medium to fast **Rest:** Nil

You will notice on my programs, that I have a combination of weights and cardio session as a workout. So, for more variety, stability, strength and challenge, include something like a BOSU® that will challenge your core muscles, as well as increase your fitness level.

1. Place the BOSU® with the flat side down. You may wish to hold a friend's hand and get used to stepping up and down initially.

2. Step up for 10 repetitions on each leg. Repeat on the other leg.

3. Make sure you are stepping right in the middle of the dome.

4.   Include your arms in a running action. This will burn more cal-
     ories and it will help you get into a rhythm with your stepping
     and stay balanced.

5.   Your sets, reps and tempo will depend on your fitness level and
     the program you are doing. Be sure to choose a program that will
     suit your level.

Tip:

If you find this too challenging, then regress to the step #DC1.

TABLE 10: LADIES' SUMMARISED TRAINING PROGRAM
– BEGINNER – BEFORE PREGNANCY

Fitness Program	Beginner	Frequency	Intensity	Time	Type	Rest Between Training Days
Cardiovascular	First 4 weeks	3-4 times per week	Light – 60% of your max heart rate	20-30 mins	Walk Bike Swim	Every other day
Resistance Training	First 4 weeks	2-3 times per week	Light – medium	30-60 mins	Dumbbells, machines with variety of Swiss ball work	Every other day
Flexibility	Part of each cardio and resistance workout	n/a	Light	20 mins –10 before, 10 after	Free/rubber band/ tubing, towel	n/a
Other	Qi Qong Yoga Pilates Feldenkrais Tai Chi	1-2 times per week	Beginner	1 hour		n/a

See my program charts for a variety of programs to suit your fitness level.

For the beginner, this is what your week should look like:

Monday	cardiovascular – 30 mins stretch – 10 mins
Tuesday	cardiovascular – 20 mins resistance – 30 mins stretch – 10 mins
Wednesday	rest day
Thursday	resistance – 60 mins stretch – 10 mins
Friday	cardiovascular – 30 mins resistance – 30 mins
Saturday	Pilates, Yoga, Qi Qong or Feldenkrais
Sunday	rest day

TABLE 11: LADIES' SUMMARISED TRAINING PROGRAM
– INTERMEDIATE – BEFORE PREGNANCY

Fitness Program	Intermediate	Frequency	Intensity	Time	Type	Rest Between Training Days
Cardiovascular	4-6 weeks	4 times per week	Medium – 70% of your max heart rate	20-60 mins	Run Bike swim	Every other day
Resistance	4-6 weeks	3-4 times per week	Medium	30-60 mins	Dumbbells, or machines with variety of Swiss ball work	Every other day
Flexibility	Part of each cardio and resistance workout	n/a	Light	20 mins – 10 before, 10 after	Free/rubber band/ tubing, towel	n/a
Other	Qi Qong Yoga Pilates Feldenkrais Tai Chi	1-2 times per week	Beginner	1 hour		n/a

For the intermediate this is what your week should look like:

Monday	resistance – 60 mins cardiovascular (run or bike) – 20 mins
Tuesday	resistance – 60 mins cardiovascular (run or bike) – 20 mins
Wednesday	rest day
Thursday	cross-training (resistance and cardiovascular) – 60 mins
Friday	Yoga or Pilates or your choice of therapeutic workout
Saturday	resistance (hard core) – 60 mins
Sunday	rest day

TABLE 12: LADIES' SUMMARISED TRAINING PROGRAM
– ADVANCED – BEFORE PREGNANCY

Fitness Program	Advanced	Frequency	Intensity	Time	Type	Rest Between Training Days
Cardiovascular	4-6 weeks	2 times per week	Medium-high – 70-80% of your max heart rate	20 mins	Run Bike swim	Every other day
Resistance	4-6 weeks	4-5 times per week	Medium-high	45-80 mins	Dumbbells, machines with variety of Swiss ball work	Every other day
Flexibility	Part of each cardio and resistance workout	n/a	Medium	20 mins – 10 before, 10 after	Free/rubber band/ tubing, towel	n/a
Other	Qi Qong Yoga Pilates Tai Chi	1-2 times per week		1 hour		n/a

For the advanced who have been training at the gym or in a group sessions, this is what your week should look like:

Monday	resistance – 60 mins cardiovascular (run or bike) – 10 mins
Tuesday	resistance – 80 mins
Wednesday	Yoga or Pilates
Thursday	resistance (hard core) – 60 mins cardiovascular (run) – 20 mins
Friday	cardiovascular (swim or run) – 20 mins (am) resistance (hard core) – 45 mins (pm)
Saturday	Yoga or Pilates
Sunday	rest day

From my experience, sometimes clients like to mix things up between some hard core group commando style classes to Bikram Yoga (heated yoga) in their week. So, there is no right or wrong way of doing things, but you need to be smart with your body and make sure you train and rest accordingly. If you are sleeping solidly and eating correctly – your body will tell you. If you are dragging a worn out and tired body due to overtraining, your body will tell you that too.

Don't allow yourself to burn out – manage yourself accordingly. Stay off stimulants like coffee or caffeinated drinks. The last thing you want is injuries!

Tip:

During your menstrual cycle, just focus on machine exercises and don't do any stability work that involves the Swiss Ball or hard core abdominal exercises. For example: Seated Chest Press Machine in place of a full push-up; Leg Press Machine rather than a bar squat. Since the uterus is swelling and shedding, the pelvic floor and lower abdominals become tender and most women get that swollen or "bloated" feel. Your stability is not as great as the rest of the month, especially in the lower back. Using a machine at this time will help you perform better quality workouts. Longer term, you are helping to protect your lower back.

EXERCISE E

SELF–MYOFASCIAL RELEASE DURING PREGNANCY

Chapter 3 "Your Fitness Program Before Pregnancy" outlined the importance and benefits of releasing muscle spasms before exercise. During pregnancy, there are only certain spots or muscles to which pressure can safely be applied, so only do the releases found in this chapter.

In this chapter you are shown how to gently release these fascia, which can play a big role in movement. For example, using a golf ball under the foot (exercise #E1) can have a lovely relaxing benefit, but it will also release spasms in the entire back area from calves, hamstrings, glutes and back muscles.

#E1

FOOT – GOLF BALL

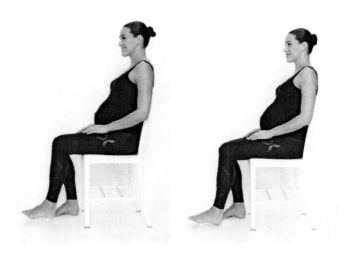

Muscles targeted: Calves, hamstrings, glutes and back.

Trimester: 1 and 2 **Intensity:** 5/10

Sets: 1 **Reps:** 1 **Hold:** 10 seconds **Rest:** nil

We often forget that our feet need just as much attention as any part of our body. One of the simple things you can do as a home treatment is use a golf ball or rolling pin and self-massage your feet. In medical terms, this is referred to as "ischemic compression", which is releasing trigger points (muscle spasms) in the small muscles or fascia in the feet.

1. Using a chair, sit in a comfortable position with the golf ball placed under one foot. Gently roll the ball up and down, sideways or in a circular movement. When you come to a tender spot, gently apply pressure and hold for 10 seconds, then roll on to another spot and hold that pressure for 10 seconds.

2. Be careful not to press too hard as you do not want to damage nerves.

3. You can spend a good five minutes on each foot.

4. The idea is to do gentle massaging, not deep pressure on nerves or muscles.

Tip:

If you do not have a golf ball, a bottle or rolling pin is a great alternative. With the rolling pin, you can also roll your foot outwards and inwards targeting the outside of the foot. This rolling will also assist in releasing tight calves, hamstrings, glutes and deep back muscles.

#E2

SHINS – TOWEL GRIP

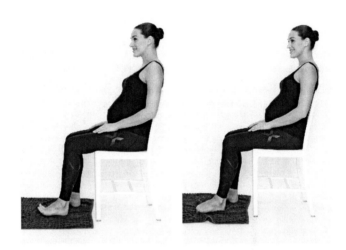

Muscles targeted: Shins (peroneal).

Trimester: 1, 2 and 3 **Intensity:** 5/10

Sets: 2 **Reps:** 10 **Hold:** N/A **Rest:** nil

The peroneal (shin) muscles can often be weak and tight.

This can prevent or hold you back from going for daily walks, as the shins can get tight and sore. One of the ways to strengthen your shins is with another self-treatment.

1. Place a towel in front of you. Place one foot on the towel. Relax your foot bending the knee at 90 degrees.

2. Gently pull your toes up, and gently gather or grip the towel under your foot.

3. Do as many grips as is comfortable for each foot. However 10 repetitions on each foot for two sets should be sufficient. If you need rest, do so for 60 seconds between sets and repeat.

4. If your toes are not gripping the towel, spraying some water on your toes should help.

Tips:

Perform after the myofascial release of golf ball under foot.

If you choose to rest between sets, you may take one foot off the floor and roll the ankle in both directions to help mobilise the ankle joint.

Caution!

If you experience pain in your foot, seek medical advice.

#E3

ILIOTIBIAL BAND – FOAM ROLLER

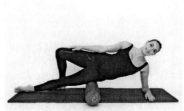
Top leg behind

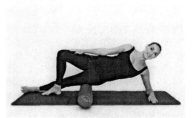
Top leg in front

Muscles targeted: Iliotibial band (ITB – side of leg fascia).

Trimester: 1 and 2 (only if comfortable) **Intensity:** 6/10

Sets: 2 **Reps:** 1 **Hold:** 15 seconds **Rest:** 10 seconds

Foam roller for the ITB (iliotibial band) is important because this band can get very tight and possibly cause the knee to roll inwards. If not treated, this can cause some knee, gluteal (buttocks/hip) weakness or even chronic knee problems.

1. From a kneeling position, place the roller on one side of your body. Lean across the roller as you support yourself on your forearm (see pic 1 & 2).

2. Lengthen the lower leg on the roller while bringing your top leg over so that the foot is positioned in front of the other knee.

3. Roll just below your hip joint, almost reaching your middle thigh. You may feel this spot is tight and tender. Start from here and work your way down the side of your thigh and almost to the knee. Maintain body alignment with legs.

4. With each spot that feels tender hold that position for 15 seconds as you breathe deeply. You may find this quite intense, but you should feel the pain and tightness ease off as the spasm slowly releases.

5. You may perform this either with your top leg behind, to get the hamstring aspect of the band, or you can place the top leg at the front of your knee and get the quadriceps aspect of the iliotibial band.

#E4

LATS AND SHOULDERS – FOAM ROLLER

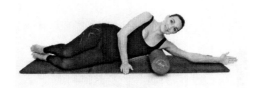

Muscles targeted: Latissimus dorsi, teres minor and teres major (back of armpit muscles).

Trimester: 1 and 2 **Intensity:** 6/10

Sets: 1 **Reps:** 1 **Hold:** 10 seconds **Rest:** 10 seconds

This will release the shoulder girdle for full range of movement.

1. Position yourself on your side with arm outstretched and foam roller under your armpit. Thumb of the extended arm is pointed up to pre-stretch the Latissimus dorsi muscle (large back muscle). Movement is minimal during this technique. Hold for 10 seconds.

2. Move up and down or side to side on the roller until you find another tender spot and hold that position for another 10 seconds.

3. Ensure your head is in a neutral position in alignment with the rest of your spine, and not dropping down or lifting up.

Tip:

If you find that the full roller is a bit tender and uncomfortable, try the half roller (pictured here), with the same technique.

Caution!

If your shoulder girdle is uncomfortable or unstable, seek medical advice.

TABLE 13: SELF-MYOFASCIAL RELEASE DURING PREGNANCY

EXERCISE	#E1 Foot – Golf Ball	#E2 Shins – Towel Grip	#E3 ITB – Foam Roller	#E4 Lats and Shoulders – Foam Roller
T1 (wk1-13)	✓	✓	✓	✓
T2 (wk14-26)	✓	✓	✓	✓
T3 (wk27-40)	NO	✓	NO	NO
Absolute Beginner	✓	✓	✓	NO
Beginner	✓	✓	✓	✓
Intermediate	✓	✓	✓	✓
Athlete	✓	✓	✓	✓
Heart Rate	Low	Low	Low	Low
Exertion Rate	Low	Low	Low	Low

Exercise F

Stretching During Pregnancy

Stretching before a workout makes your muscles supple and ready for activity and movement. Pregnancy is not the time to work on increasing flexibility. Your stretching should be mild, enabling you to experience full range of movement without experiencing joint pain, tension or stiffness.

Stretching is also a great way to relax and reduce tension or stress.

Avoid any stretches where your head is lower than your heart (a traditional caution given to pregnant yoga practitioners as in "downward dog").

The hormone Relaxin is another contributor to lower back pain. During pregnancy, the hormone Relaxin is present at 10 times its normal concentration in the female body. Relaxin is beneficial in the sense that its function (as you may gather from the name) is to relax the joints in the pelvis so the baby has room to pass through the birth canal. Unfortunately, Relaxin also causes abnormal motion in many other joints of the body, causing inflammation and pain.[37] Remember not to overstretch, but simply continue with the static (holding) stretches outlined below.

In these stretches, I suggest holding each for 10 to 20 seconds, however if you feel you need to hold a particular stretch for longer or do an extra set, that is fine as long as you take care not to bounce as you stretch and avoid a feeling of pulling in your muscles or joints.

During pregnancy, it's all about being active, strong and getting your body ready for the delivery of the baby. Following the birth, you should recover more quickly to be strong enough for resuming normal training.

A Special Note to Athletes: Even though this book does not contain a lot of detail specifically for athletes, who are generally quite flexible,

---

37 http://health.discovery.com/centers/pregnancy/backpain.html

you should note that during pregnancy, stretching needs to be regressed due to the hormone Relaxin.

#F1

CALF – WALL

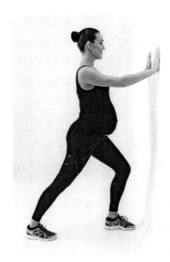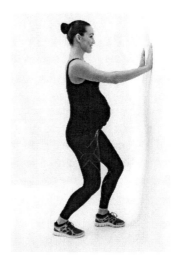

Muscles targeted: Gastrocnemius (calves).

Trimester: 1, 2 and 3

Sets: 1 **Reps:** 1 **Hold:** 20 seconds

1. Stand in a split stance near a wall, doorway or large stationary object.

2. Bring one leg forward for support; use your upper body to lean against the wall. Your neck, spine, pelvis and outstretched leg (back leg) should form one straight line. Keep back foot flat, with toes pointed to the front.

3. Gently draw your lower abdomen inward toward your spine.

4. Lean towards the wall with your chest and hips, until you feel the calf stretch in your back leg.

5. Stop movement when slight tension is felt and hold for 20 seconds.

6. You may have feet that pronate (roll inwards) – to avoid this, press your little toe on the floor to stretch the calf properly. If one of your calves is tighter than the other, you may need to stretch that side again or hold your stretch position a little longer.

Tip:

If you experience some sciatic nerve pain throughout pregnancy, then during your calf stretch, pressing your little toe down to the floor is beneficial. (Sciatica is nerve pain from irritation of the sciatic nerve. The pain is typically felt from the low back (lumbar area) to behind the thigh and radiating down below the knee).

#F2

ACHILLES – WALL OR CHAIR VERSION

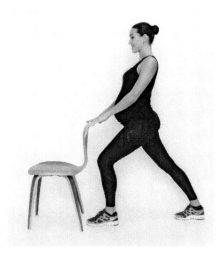

Muscles targeted: Achilles and soleus (lower portion of the calf muscles and tendons).

Trimester: 1, 2 and 3

Sets: 1 **Reps:** 1 **Hold:** 20 seconds

The soleus (muscle below the calf) is always tight and often neglected. The soleus is stretched with a minor adjustment to the standing calf stretch. This will help you gain proper function in squatting and walking.

1. Stand in the calf stretch position. Gently bend the back knee while keeping both heels down to the floor.

2. Hold this position for 10 to 20 seconds.

3. Swap over to the other side, always doing an extra repetition on the tighter leg.

Tip:

Women wearing high heels for prolonged periods will benefit from this stretch, as these heels cause the calves and soleus muscles to become very tight and short.

#F3

HAMSTRING – STANDING OR SEATED

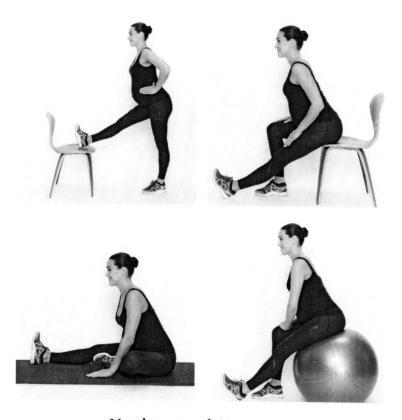

Muscles targeted: Hamstrings.

Trimester: 1, 2 and 3

Sets: 1 **Reps:** 1 **Hold:** 20 seconds

Hamstrings play a big role in back care. Since these muscles are much like the calves – short and tight, it is important to increase flexibility and mobility around the hip joint. For many seated at a desk job for the majority of the day, the hamstrings are flexed for prolonged periods.

1. If you are accustomed to a standing hamstring stretch, continue using that version. You may also choose to try the chair or ball version – see which feels the most comfortable for you.

2. Using either a Swiss ball or chair, position one leg in front with the heel down and toes flexed (pulled towards your body).

3. Bend or flex forward at the hips until you feel the first resistance barrier and hold for 20 seconds. Keep your back tall with a curvature in your lower spine and gently lean forward. Repeat on the other side.

Progression:

From a static stretch, you may progress onto dynamic stretch by moving the toes forward (away from you) as if you are toe-tapping the floor and then moving the toes backwards to achieve a great stretch throughout the hamstrings.

#F4

INNER THIGH – KNEELING, SEATED OR SWISS BALL

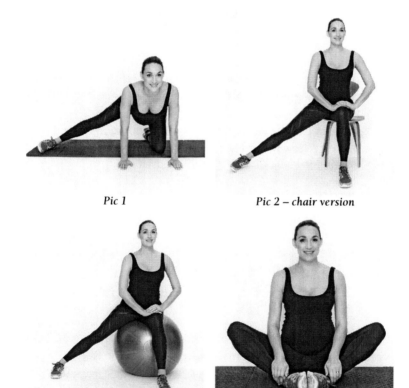

Pic 1   Pic 2 – chair version

Pic 3 – ball version   Pic 4

Muscles targeted: Inner thigh.

Trimester: 1, 2 and 3

Sets: 1 **Reps:** 1 **Hold:** 20 seconds

Your inner thigh muscles play an important role in hip mobility, strength and flexibility. These muscles are consistently ignored and neglected, leaving many women with constant tightness and soreness around their hips and lower back.

1. Start by positioning yourself on all fours (pic 1).

2. Make sure your body is lengthened while keeping the curvature in your lower back.

3. Take one leg straight out to the side, level with the hip (pic 1).

4. Have your foot turned in, so it is flat on the floor. This is an important stretch as sometimes it correlates with tight outside hips (buttocks – gluteus medius and/or minimus) on the same side.

5. Find your comfortable spot, as sometimes you may need to move your body forward or back to set yourself up for a good comfortable stretch.

6. Pic 2 and 3 – Sit on a chair or Swiss ball, with a tall posture, both feet in front while maintaining the curvature in your lower back.

7. Take one leg out to the side with the foot planted on the floor or rolled in – whichever is more comfortable.

8. Flex the other leg at 90 degrees at the knee.

9. Lean forward on your front (bent) knee and you will feel your hip opening up nicely into a lovely stretch.

10. Make sure that your knee and foot are aligned and tracking directly over the second toe.

11. Hold for 10-20 seconds. Repeat other side.

12. Pic 4 – Sit on the floor with both knees bent and feet together. Allow your knees to fall to each side and hold the stretch to for a comfortable time. You can also do some breathing in and some pelvic floor contractions.

Progression:

From chair version to ball or floor version.

Regression:

If there is pubic symphysis (the instability of the pelvic joint due to the hormone Relaxin sometimes causing strange and painful sensations in this region), please see your physiotherapist or try the chair version.

#F5

PIRIFORMIS – HIP STRETCH ON THE SWISS BALL OR CHAIR

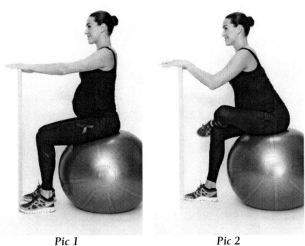

Pic 1   Pic 2

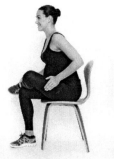

Pic 3

Muscles targeted: Piriformis (hip and gluteal area).

Trimester: 1, 2 and 3

Sets: 2 Reps: 1 Hold: 10-20 seconds

Piriformis stretch on the ball is one of the most effective stretches for the hip and glutes. The sciatic nerve runs through this muscle, hence this stretch should be a priority on your list. This stretch will release the tightness and stiffness in the hip and glutes area.

1. Position the Swiss ball close to a stable object.

2. Sitting tall on the ball, lift one leg and place the ankle on the opposite thigh (pic 2).

3. Breathe in; as you breathe out gently bend forward, maintaining long upper body and neutral curvature in lumbar (lower) spine.

4. Hold this position for 20 seconds, and repeat the other side.

If you do not have a ball, the chair version is just as effective (pic 3).

Caution!

If there is any inner thigh or hip discomfort, seek medical advice.

#F6

QUADRICEPS – STANDING OR LYING DOWN

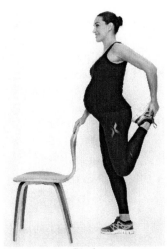

Pic 1

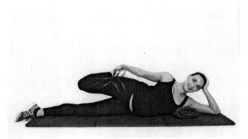

Pic 2

Muscles targeted: Quadriceps (front thigh) and hips.

Trimester: 1, 2 and 3

Sets: 1 **Reps:** 1 **Hold:** 20 seconds

One of the most common stretches is the standing quad stretch. Flexible quad and hip flexor muscles are important for hip and back function.

1. Supporting yourself on a wall or stable object, bend one leg at the knee and bring your heel towards your glutes. Feel the stretch in the front thigh, while gently softening and bending the other knee.

2. Contract or squeeze your glutes and you should feel extra stretch or opening in that hip. Hold the tension and stretch in the thigh muscle for 20 seconds.

3. Release and change to the other leg.

4. The floor version may be more comfortable for you as you progress from T1 to T2. Lie on your side and support your head with a rolled up towel. Use the top arm to bring your heel towards your glutes.

5. Maintain good body alignment. Hold this stretch for 20 seconds. You can repeat this if you wish, as this stretch can be quite relaxing.

Tips:

Make sure that the supported leg is slightly bent at the knee (pic 1), taking pressure off the locked knee and the back.

If you are not able to do this stretch in the standing position, then lie down on the floor and perform the same. You should find that the floor version has less pressure on the knees.

#F7

HIP FLEXOR – STANDING

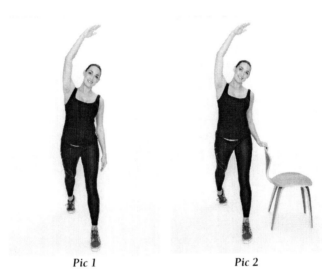

Pic 1   Pic 2

Muscles targeted: Psoas (hip flexor), quadratus lumborum (lower back) and obliques (waist – front and back).

Trimester: 1, 2 and 3

Sets: 1 **Reps:** 1 **Hold:** 10 seconds

You will find that all of the muscles around your hip will become tighter as your pregnancy progresses. It is very important to stretch these muscles, not only for your posture but so that squatting and lunging, during exercise and daily life, becomes easier.

1. Stand tall in a split stance position with both knees slightly bent, lifting your back heel off the floor.

2. Raise one arm up towards the ceiling.

3. Maintaining your tall posture, take a breath in and as you breathe out, reach up with the arm. While breathing out, lean over to the opposite side in a controlled and relaxed manner.

4. You should feel your hip and waist stretching. Hold this stretch for 10 seconds. Your breathing will greatly assist you as you are relaxing through your stretch.

Tips:

If you need some support, choose the chair version shown in pic 2.

Do not over stretch with the arm up or lock up in your lower back.

#F8

HIP FLEXOR STRETCH – KNEELING

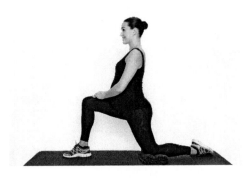

Muscles targeted: Hip flexors and quadriceps (front of thighs).

Trimester: 1, 2 and 3

Sets: 1 **Reps:** 1 **Hold:** 10-20 seconds

Trimesters: This stretch will mostly benefit you in T1 and T2.

1. From a kneeling position, take one leg forward in front of your body. *Make sure you are at 90 degrees in the front knee*, avoiding pressure in either knee or leg.

2. Your shoulders should be directly over your hips, and *DO NOT lean forward* or you will lose the effect of the stretch.

3. Tuck your glutes under, as if you are tilting your tailbone underneath. Hold that position and slowly lean forward with your hips feeling the stretch and opening of your hip.

4. Extend your body to a full upright position and hold for 10 seconds.

5. Swap to the other side.

Tip:

If you need more comfort, it may be a good idea to fold a towel or place a cushion under your knee.

#F9

SIDE LEG

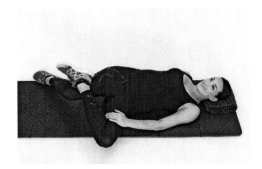

Muscles targeted: ITB – Iliotibial band/fascia.

Trimester: 1 and 2

Sets: 1 **Reps:** 1 **Hold:** 10 seconds

There are a number of ITB stretches. This version, together with the foam roller release, is a good combination.

1. Lie on your back with your palms out to each side and both knees comfortably bent.

2. Place one foot on the outside of the opposite knee.

3. Gently bring that knee down towards the floor, feeling the hip and side of leg being stretched. Hold for 10 seconds. Repeat on the other side.

Tip:

Relax your hips and inner thighs.

Caution!

If you experience discomfort when performing this stretch, avoid it.

#F10

LOWER BACK AND WAIST – SWISS BALL

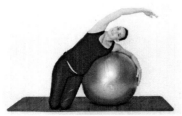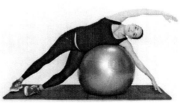

Pic 1
Mostly supported on the floor

Pic 2
Split position – legs apart

Muscles targeted: Quadratus lumborum (lower back), obliques (waist- - front and back) and latissimus dorsi (upper back).

Trimester: 1 and 2

Sets: 1 **Reps:** 1 **Hold:** 10-20 seconds

This stretch would mostly benefit you in T1 and T2. If you are not accustomed to stretching with the ball, then I would only suggest it in T1 and continue with the stretch as in pic 1. Be your own judge of safety during T2 – make sure you are stable on the ball.

1. Start by sitting sideways and hugging the Swiss ball with the arm closest to the ball. Use your other arm to extend up and over your head. This will give you a nice waist stretch.

2. Use the first stretch where you are mostly supported on the floor, and then progress to split position (legs apart) and roll to a full stretch.

3. Once you feel comfortable with the position of the ball and your waist being right in the middle of the ball, straighten your top

leg while keeping your foot on the floor and allow your top arm to fall naturally above your head, so that your body makes one straight line from foot to knee, to hip and shoulder.

4. Keep your lower leg bent for support.

5. To return to the starting position, slowly lower your hips down to the floor and repeat on the other side.

#F11

CHEST – SWISS BALL OR STANDING

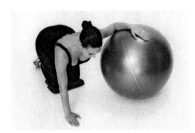
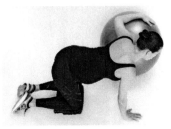
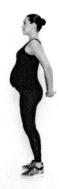

Muscles targeted: Pectorals (chest) and shoulders.

Trimester: 1, 2 and 3

Sets: 1 **Reps:** 1 **Hold:** 20 seconds

1. From a 4-point kneeling position, place one arm and hand on top of the ball, bending the elbow at 90 degrees.

2. Make sure that you are not shrugging with your shoulders, but rather pulling your shoulder blades in towards your spine. Knees are hip-width apart, keeping the curvature in your lower back and neck.

3. Slowly allow the body to relax, dropping the chest towards the floor. Look down to the floor the whole time, so that your neck does not hyperextend. Hold for 10-20 seconds.

Standing version (without ball)

If you do not have a ball, the standing version is another relaxing way to stretch your chest.

1. Stand tall with knees slightly bent and lift your pelvic floor muscles. Take both arms back and interlock your fingers. Lift your ribcage, breathing in and out as you do, open out the chest and hold the stretch for 20 seconds.

Tip:

Ball version – You can adjust the arm position forward and back to get different aspects of the chest stretch. Also, add mild pressure on the ball with your arm, with normal breathing.

#F12

LATISSIMUS – SWISS BALL

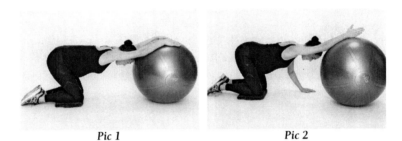

Pic 1   Pic 2

Muscles targeted: Latissimus dorsi (long back muscles) and shoulders.

Trimester: 1, 2 and 3

Sets: 1 **Reps:** 1 **Hold:** 20 seconds

The latissimus dorsi muscle is one of the largest back muscles. It works together with your gluteus for stability and posture.

1. From a kneeling position, extend both arms on top of the ball (pic 1). Just being in this position may be sufficient, however if you wish to feel a more intense stretch, lean back towards your heels. Alternatively, you can remain kneeling and feeling the chest gently drop down towards the floor. Maintain a normal breathing pattern for a few breaths as you enjoy the stretch.

2. To stretch individual sides, support yourself on one arm keeping it in line with the shoulder, while outstretching the other on top of the ball. Hold that position for 10 seconds and then gently push the arm further away from you so that you feel the side or latissimus dorsi muscle (armpit area and lower back) stretch.

Tip:

With every breath, try to relax your chest and back, feeling yourself relax towards the floor.

Progression:

Sit back on your heels and roll the ball side to side in a slow and controlled manner.

#F13

BACK – SWISS BALL

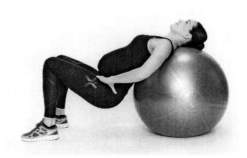

Muscles targeted: Thoracic (upper, mid and lower back).

Trimester: 1 and 2 (only if comfortable)

Sets: 1 **Reps:** 1 **Hold:** 10 seconds

One of the important stretches is the thoracic stretch. Our daily posture requires sitting in a forward and slouched position. Therefore, we need to take extra care of our back. Stretching in this manner may alleviate some back pain and be relaxing.

This stretch may or may not be comfortable for you. Try it and, if you feel the benefits, continue.

1. From a seated position, slowly walk forward until you feel your lower back is wrapped around the ball. Your feet should be in line with your knees at 90 degrees.

2. Make sure your head is supported on the ball the whole time while you enjoy the stretch for 10 seconds. To return, tuck your chin in and roll yourself up as if you are doing an abdominal

crunch. Walk your feet backwards towards the ball and slowly rolling up to starting position.

Tip:

If you enjoy this stretch, you can do it every day.

Caution!

If you find your upper and/or lower back is stiff, please do not do this exercise.

#F14

NECK – BACK

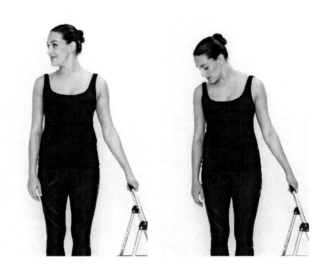

Muscles targeted: Upper trapezius (neck muscles).

Trimester: 1, 2 and 3

Sets: 1 **Reps:** 1 **Hold:** 20 seconds

Almost every woman I have trained has been tight in this area. As you progress in your pregnancy, sleeping will become uncomfortable, and your neck and back of your shoulder blades will experience some discomfort. It's import-ant that you do this stretch daily. Consider even doing a couple of these stretches while at your desk.

1. Hold on to a steady object such as a bar, with your left hand. Keep your arm straight, so that you feel the shoulder has no movement.

2. Gently turn your head sideways to the right. Hold the position for 20 seconds.

3. Bring your head back to neutral position, and this time on the same side, turn your head 45 degrees and drop your chin towards your chest. Your head must be nice and relaxed in order to feel the stretch in the back of your neck. Breathe in; as you breathe out feel the stretch. Hold for 15 to 20 seconds. Repeat on the opposite side.

Tips:

In order to get the most from your stretch, you should have a tall posture with your shoulders relaxed and pushed downwards.

Gently place your opposite hand on top of your head. ***Do not pull*** on your head or neck. You may repeat this for a second set if you are experiencing tightness in this area.

#F15

NECK – SIDE AND FRONT

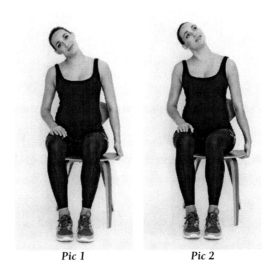

Pic 1   Pic 2

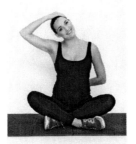

Pic 3

Muscles targeted: Scalenes (side and front of neck).

Trimester: 1, 2 and 3

Sets: 1 **Reps:** 1 **Hold:** 20 seconds

These muscles are often neglected in our stretching routine. They can often become tight, as they are attached to the first rib under your clavicle (collarbone). If this is a tight muscle for you, it will prevent you from performing effective push-ups and will create a feeling of tightness or stiffness in the neck. Also your diaphragmatic breathing will be improved – which is important for pelvic floor and core muscle contraction.

1. Sit tall on a chair keeping good posture. Reach down with your left hand and grab the side of chair to anchor the shoulder girdle.

2. Gently tilt your head to the right side, making sure you are looking up.

3. Rotate the head and chin looking up. Feel the front part of your neck feeling the stretch. Hold the stretch for 20 seconds.

4. Pic 3 shows the seated floor version. Placing one bent arm behind your lower back will give you a greater and relaxed stretch. Placing the hand on the outside of your head, adds a comfortable stretch.

Tip:

To maximise your stretch, place two fingers of your opposite hand on the forehead. Remain in the same posture with anchored shoulder. Breathe in; gently push your forehead into your fingers and vice versa. Hold the tension for 5 seconds and relax, feeling the stretch intensify. Repeat on the other side.

#F16

NECK – BACK

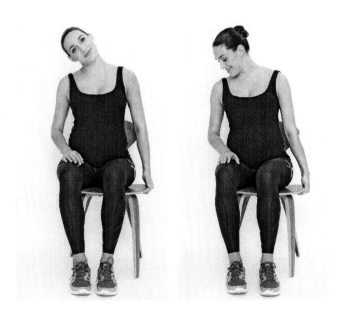

Muscles targeted: Levator scapulae (long back of the neck muscles).

Trimester: 1, 2 and 3

Sets: 1 **Reps:** 1 **Hold:** 20 seconds

This muscle begins from the second vertebrae in the neck/spine and attaches just above the shoulder blade. It is the most common cause of neck pain. Consequently, the levator scapulae take and carry the entire load of any kind of stress, bad posture or stiffness around the neck. This is one of the muscles that you must not trigger point, or press on the shoulder to release tightness. So stretching is the best thing that you can do to release tightness.

1. Sitting on a chair, take your left hand and grip to the side of the chair. Gently turn your head to 45 degrees and gently lower your chin towards your armpit or chest.

2. Feel the stretch from the base of the skull all the way down to your shoulder blade. Hold the stretch for 20 seconds.

Tips:

If you are tall and have long arms and legs, you will benefit more from sitting on a bench, as your long arms need to extend to the back of the bench to get a grip on the side/back of the bench, so that the shoulder does not move during your stretch.

You can place the opposite hand on top of your head, and gently hold while you feel a slight tension into your hand. Hold for 5 counts and release. Repeat a few times and feel the neck stretching.

#F17

BACK AND BREATHING STRETCH – SWISS BALL

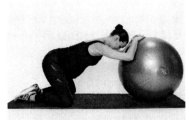 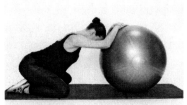

Muscles targeted: All back muscles.

Trimester: 1, 2 and 3

Sets: 1 **Reps:** 1 **Hold:** 20 seconds

1. From a kneeling position, place your knees wider than your hips. Arms are bent at the elbows and relaxed on top of the Swiss ball. Lean back towards your heels and feel the upper and lower back relax into your stretch.

2. Just being in this position may encourage you to do some breathing exercises to prepare you for labour.

3. Allow your lower back to relax and your chest and shoulders to drop towards the floor.

Tip:

With every breath, lift and contract your pelvic floor muscles. Relax your chest and back, feeling yourself relax towards the floor.

TABLE 14: STRETCHING DURING PREGNANCY – ALL TRIMESTERS

EXERCISE	T1 (wk1-13)	T2 (wk14-26)	T3 (wk27-40)	Absolute Beginner	Beginner	Inter-mediate	Athlete	Heart Rate	Exertion Rate
#F1 Calf – Wall	✓	✓	✓	✓	✓	✓	20 secs	Low	Low
#F2 Achilles – Wall/Chair Version	✓	✓	✓	No	✓	✓	20 secs	Low	Low
#F3 Hamstrings	✓	✓	Pic 2	✓	✓	✓	20 secs	Low	Low
#F4 Inner Thigh	✓		Pic 2	✓	✓	✓	20 secs	Low	Low
#F5 Piriformis – Hip	✓	✓	Pic 3	✓	✓	✓	20 secs	Low	Low
#F6 Quadriceps	✓	✓	Pic 2	✓	✓	✓	20 secs	Low	Low
#F7 Hip Flexor – Standing	✓	✓	✓	No	No	✓	20 secs	Low	Low
#F8 Hip Flexor – Kneeling	✓	✓	✓	✓	✓	Pic 2 for athletes T1 only *	10-20 secs	Low	Low
#F9 Side Leg	✓	No	No	No	✓	✓	10 secs	Low	Low
#F10 Lower Back and Waist	✓	✓	No	No	✓	✓	20 secs	Low	Low
#F11 Chest	✓	✓	✓	Standing only	Standing	✓	20 secs	Low	Low
#F12 Latissimus	✓	✓	✓	No	No	✓	20 secs	Low	Low
#F13 Back	✓	✓	✓	No	No	✓	20 secs	Low	Low
#F14 Neck – Back	✓	✓	✓	✓	✓	✓	20 secs	Low	Low
#F15 Neck – Side and Front	✓	✓	✓	No	No	✓	20 secs	Low	Low
#F16 Neck – Back	✓	✓	✓	✓	✓	✓	20 secs	Low	Low
#F17 Back and Breathing	✓	✓	✓	✓	✓	✓	20-60 secs	Low	Low

*Hip Flexor on the ball can only be used by advanced people or athletes within the first few weeks of pregnancy. If you continue to do this stretch, it creates too much pressure on the front of the hip and knee ligaments, tendons and joints, potentially causing injury.

EXERCISE G

MOBILITY AND STABILITY DURING PREGNANCY – THE SECRET TO A STRONG AND STABLE PELVIS

Mobility is not the same as flexibility. Mobility is your range of motion under specific circumstances. It focuses on creating stability, smoothness and freedom of movement as opposed to flexibility, which is about increasing range of motion about a joint and is non-specific. For example, by mobilising the pelvis in a rocking motion or a circular motion, we allow the muscles to loosen up around the hips and back, enabling movement to become more fluid and functional. This in turn, improves the stability of the pelvis and hips in performing such motions as squatting and lunging.

I CANNOT STRESS THE IMPORTANCE OF THESE EXERCISES ENOUGH! Even if you choose to do only these during your pregnancy, together with some comfortable cardio work, you will still benefit greatly. Mobility and stability exercises will bring more body-awareness and help you to focus on strengthening your hips and back, while lengthening the lower back muscles.

In Group C *Mobility and Stability for Before and After Pregnancy – The Secret to a Strong and Stable Pelvis*, we performed strength-based exercises to strengthen muscles around the pelvis and internal core muscles. In this chapter, you will notice the exercises have more of a warm up type movement e.g. pelvic tilts. While some of the exercises may be the same as in Group C *Mobility and Stability for Before and After Pregnancy – The Secret to a Strong and Stable Pelvis,* be careful to note which exercises are only suitable for certain trimesters e.g. lower body rotation is only for T1 and T2.

The following exercises are easy, gentle and therapeutic. You can do these as a complete workout if you wish, performing them a couple of times a week. You will feel amazing afterwards!

Description of Pelvic Tilts:

Anterior Pelvic Tilt: Hip bones or pelvis is tilted forward in a standing or sitting position – glutes are sticking out creating a curve in your lower back. Posture is upright and tall.

Posterior Pelvic Tilt: Hip bones or pelvis is tilted backwards in a standing or sitting position – glutes are tucked under as though you are bringing your hips closer to your ribs. Posture is upright while creating a flat back.

Lateral Tilt: Hip bones or pelvis are tilted side to side. Posture is upright and tall.

#G1

LATERAL PELVIC TILT – SIDE TO SIDE TILT

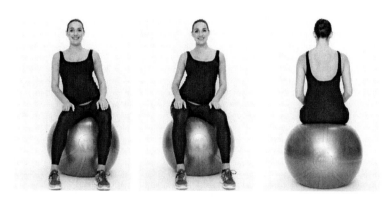

Muscles targeted: Muscles around the pelvis, e.g. hips and lower back.

Trimester: 1, 2 and 3 **Intensity:** Low

Sets: 2 **Reps:** 20 **Tempo:** Slow **Rest:** 30 seconds

Pelvic tilts are a great way to mobilise and stretch the lumbar (lower back) region.

1. Sit on the Swiss ball with good posture, your feet a little wider than shoulder-width apart and knees bent at 90 degrees.

2. Place your hands on your thighs, and maintain a tall posture and a neutral curvature in your lumbar (lower back) area.

3. Brace the lower abdominal and pelvic floor muscles, while maintaining normal breathing. Gently tilt sideways, bringing the hip and ribs closer together – close the gap at the waist, while stretching the lower back on the opposite side.

4. Complete 10 to each side. Repeat for 2 sets with 30 seconds rest between each set.

Tip:

Make sure you have your feet wider than your hips. If you slouch, this is incorrect and you will not feel your lower back stretch. Be sure to lift your ribcage as you begin.

Regression:

Make smaller movements from side to side.

#G2

ANTERIOR AND POSTERIOR PELVIC TILT – FRONT AND BACK TILT

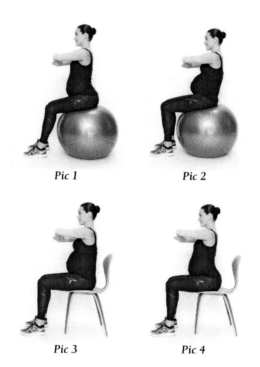

Pic 1   Pic 2

Pic 3   Pic 4

Muscles targeted: Pelvis, hips and lower back.

Trimester: 1, 2 and 3 **Intensity:** Low

Sets: 2 **Reps:** 20 **Tempo:** Slow **Rest:** 30 seconds

If you have a desk job, run around after your children picking up things off the floor or load and offload shopping, your lower back will be either locking up or the muscles tensing up. This is one way of mobilising and releasing that tension.

- **Anterior tilt** – glutes pushed backwards-creating arch in lower back (pic 1).
- **Posterior tilt** – glutes tucked under, flattening your lower back out (pic 2).

1. Assume the same position as for the side-to-side tilt.

2. In the photo, the model's arms are folded in front of her, so you can see the distinct tilt. When you are doing this, keep your hands on your thighs, not folded in front (pic 3 & 4).

3. Breathe in diaphragmatically; lift the pelvic floor muscles away from the ball first. Maintain the contraction while you are tilting your buttocks under – (posterior tilt) followed by tilting your pelvis backwards (anterior pelvic tilt).

4. Continue front and back tilting 20 times (front 10 tilts and back 10 tilts). You can do this at any time of the day you wish.

Tip:

Your first set can be used for mobilising the lumbar (lower back) region. If you wish to concentrate on your core and pelvic floor contraction, hold the posterior pelvic tilt (tilt your glutes under) with a pelvic lift for 10 seconds. The chair version can be done at work or at any other time you are seated.

Progression:

On the Swiss Ball, **circle** 10 times in one direction and 10 times in the other. This allows the pelvis and the tailbone region to relax and mobilise.

#G3

LATERAL PELVIC TILT – KNEELING POSITION (ALTERNATIVE TO BALL VERSION)

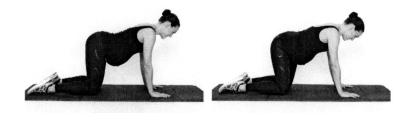

Muscles targeted: Lower back, pelvis and hips.

Trimester: 1, 2 and 3 **Intensity:** Low

Sets: 2 **Reps:** 20 **Tempo:** Slow **Rest:** 30 seconds

There are many lower backstretches, and this is one of the more comfortable as you do not have to lie on your back in order to stretch your lower back.

1. Take the 4-point kneeling position (see exercise #C6). Knees are under hips and hands under shoulders, without locking your elbows.

2. Breathing naturally in a relaxed way, gently tilt your hips to the right side of your body. This stretches your lower back on the left side.

3. Maintaining natural breathing, gently tilt your hips to the left side of your body. This stretches your lower back on the right side.

4. Repeat this as many times as comfortable, aiming for a total of 20 repetitions. If you wish to hold the stretch longer, you may do so.

5. Rest for 30 seconds and repeat for the second set.

#G4

RUSSIAN TWIST – SWISS BALL

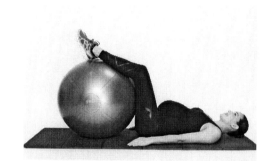

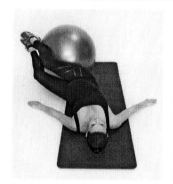 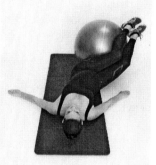

Muscles targeted: Lower back, hips, core and obliques.

Trimester: 1 and 2 **Intensity:** Low to moderate

Sets: 1-3 **Reps:** 10 **Tempo:** 3:1:3 **Rest:** 60 seconds

1. Lie on your back with the Swiss ball under your calves. Upper body (neck and shoulders) is relaxed with palms down and out to 45 degrees.

2. Position the ball close to your hamstrings and calves.

3. Breathe in diaphragmatically. As you breathe out, gently roll the ball to the left side of your body. Take another breath in. As you breathe out, roll the ball back to your starting position. Repeat this to the right side with the same breathing pattern. This is one repetition.

4. Repeat this for 1 to 3 sets, turning on your left side for 60 seconds as a rest period.

5. You will most likely be able to do this for both T1 and T2, which is fine. Listen to your body and only do what you comfortably can.

Tip:

As you go over to each side, keep the opposite shoulder on the floor at all times. This will help to mobilise and stretch your lower back.

To begin with, allow your legs to go only as low as is comfortable.

Caution!

Beyond 16 weeks you should avoid lying on your back for prolonged periods, due to the danger of restricting blood flow to your heart.

#G5

MUSCLE ENERGY RELEASE

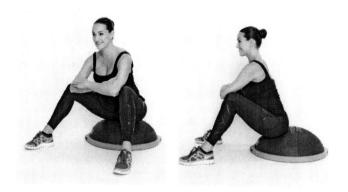

Muscles targeted: Core muscles, pelvis, inner thigh and hips.

Trimester: 1, 2 and 3 (only if comfortable) **Intensity:** Low

Sets: 1-2 **Reps:** 10 **Tempo:** Controlled **Rest:** 60 seconds

The purpose of this exercise is to both mentally and physically help you develop good breathing patterns and to prepare your pelvis for natural delivery. This is a 2-fold exercise which comfortably stretches the inner thighs and contracts the pelvic floor muscles as well as strengthens the pelvis and outer thighs.

1. The model pictured here is sitting on a dome called a BOSU®; however you can use a beanbag or a large cushion to do this exercise.

2. If you are sitting on a beanbag, adjust your position to ensure your hips are at an even level; a lumpy beanbag will not give you a balanced sitting position.

3. This is a great muscle energy technique, which involves voluntary muscle contractions for a count of 5-10 seconds. It is used for joint mobilisation and for stretching tense muscles.

4. Remember the tension created is about 5-10%. Do not push or pull hard. It's a mild sensation throughout.

Inner Thigh

1. Position yourself with legs wide apart, so that your tummy is comfortable and you are able to place each elbow on the inside of each knee.

2. Lifting your pelvic floor muscles first, and only then contract your inner thighs by gently pushing against your elbows.

3. Hold for 5 - 10 counts. Maintain normal breathing in between each repetition. Repeat 10 times.

Outer Thigh

1. The same technique is used for the outer thigh, except the elbows are wrapped around the outside of each knee, and the pushing will be external (outside) for 5-10 counts. If you find the elbows uncomfortable, you may place your hands on the outside of each knee instead.

Tip:

When lifting your pelvic floor muscles, make sure you only have a maximum of 20% contraction. Contracting more than that, you will lose the effectiveness and coordination with lower abdominal muscles. Over-activation of the pelvic floor muscles is not advisable.

Caution!

If you are suffering with pubic symphysis (the instability of the pelvic joint due to the hormone Relaxin sometimes causing strange and painful sensations in this region), do not do this exercise and seek medical attention.

#G6

HIP EXTENSION WITH FEET ON THE SWISS BALL

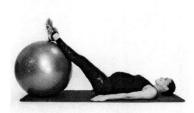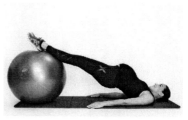

Muscles targeted: Gluteus, hamstrings, hips and core.

Trimester: 1 and 2 (only if comfortable) **Intensity:** Low to moderate

Sets: 1-3 **Reps:** 8-12 **Tempo:** 2:2:2 **Rest:** 60 seconds

This is an excellent exercise to warm up the glutes and hip muscles, especially after your pelvis has been mobilised with mobilisation or stretches. Your squats will be more effective and you will feel stronger after doing these.

1. Lie on your back with heels and calves shoulder-width apart and comfortably on the Swiss ball. Make sure your feet are in the middle of the ball. Place your palms down and out to 45 degrees for support.

2. Lift your hips up in 2 counts and stabilise. Hold for 2 counts and come down for 2 counts.

3. Continue this lift for a maximum of 12 repetitions in total and rest for 60 seconds on your left side to recover.

4. You may do one set, just to "wake up" the glutes and hips muscles, or you can do 3 sets to gain maximum benefit.

Regression:

Move the ball closer to you and place your calves on the ball instead of the heels.

#G7

HIP EXTENSION WITH FEET ON THE FLOOR

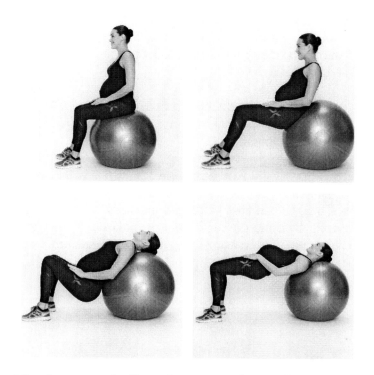

Muscles targeted: Glutes, hamstrings, hips and lower back.

Trimester: 1, 2 and 3 (only if comfortable) **Intensity:** Low

Sets: 1-3 **Reps:** 10 **Tempo:** 3:2:3 **Rest:** 60 seconds

1. From a seated position, walk yourself forward until you are in a comfortable position. Support your head and shoulders in the centre of the ball. Place your hands on your hips and stabilise.

2. Breathe in through your diaphragm. As you breathe out draw your bellybutton in towards your spine. Lift pelvic floor muscles, and only then gently lift your hips/glutes towards the ceiling.

3. Ensure you stay lengthened with a neutral lower back curvature and do not hyperextend (lifting your hips up too high or making a huge lower back arch).

4. Squeeze your glutes and feel the hips opening out. Normal tempo is down for 3 counts, come up in 2 counts and hold for 3. During T1 and T2, you can hold for 5 counts and really focus on contracting the glutes. Keep feet flat pushing through your heels and not through your toes.

5. Repeat going down and up in a controlled manner. Remember to breathe in your normal breathing pattern and still contract into your pelvic floor muscles.

Tip:

Do not roll the ball backwards and forwards, this defeats the purpose of getting maximum strength from the glutes. If you do not have a ball or you are not used to using one, refer to the home program for the floor version.

#G8

HIP EXTENSION WITH FEET ON THE FLOOR – MEDICINE BALL OR TOWEL BETWEEN LEGS

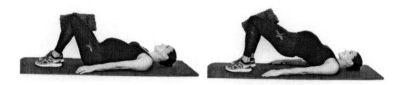

Muscles targeted: Gluteus, hamstrings, inner thigh and hips.

Trimester: 1, 2 and 3 (only if comfortable) **Intensity:** Low

Sets: 1-3 **Reps:** 10 **Tempo:** 3:2:3 **Rest:** 60 seconds

In my experience, there is very little if anything done to exercise and strengthen the inner thigh muscles for pregnant women. However, this is a very important area because weak hip muscles must work together with the inner thighs.

Most women would like to improve the tone of their inner thigh muscles. I encourage you to take few minutes to do this exercise. I guarantee that if you do it properly, your legs will feel the benefit after just a couple of sets.

1. Bend your knees at 45 degrees and place a large folded towel (or if you have a small medicine ball e.g. 1kg) between your knees or your thighs.

2. Breathe in; as you breathe out, draw your pelvic floor muscles up and deep abdominal wall in.

3. Push through your heels and lift your glutes off the floor in 3 counts, squeezing the towel and holding for 2 counts at the same time. Release in 3 counts while lowering down to the floor.

4. Repeat this for a total of 10 repetitions and rest on your left side for 1 minute. Repeat this again for another 2 sets.

Tip:

During T1 you can hold the contraction for up to 5 seconds.

#G9

BUTTOCK SQUEEZE – WITH TUBE

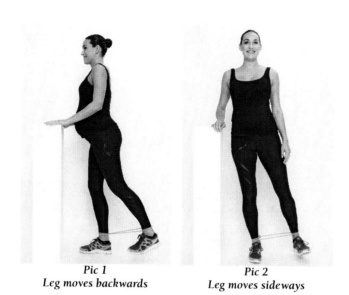

Pic 1
Leg moves backwards

Pic 2
Leg moves sideways

Muscles targeted: Gluteus and hips.

Trimester: 1 and 2 **Intensity:** Low to moderate

Sets: 1-3 **Reps:** 5-10 **Tempo:** 2:1:2 **Rest:** 60 seconds

1. This exercise can be performed either with or without a rubber tube (picture uses tube). If you haven't done this exercise before, perform it without the tube. When choosing a rubber tube, select one that is about hip-width apart.

2. Step into the tube and position it around your ankles. Stand supported against a wall with feet shoulder-width apart. Slightly bend the left leg at the knee. Before you begin moving your opposite leg, lift your pelvic floor muscles and draw in your lower abdomen. Keep your hips still and aligned with the shoulders.

There should be no movement in the hips while performing the leg lift.

3. To work your gluteus maximus (pic 1), extend your right leg backwards until you feel your corresponding glute tighten up. Do not swing the leg, as this will compromise your posture.

4. To work your gluteus medius (hip muscle - pic 2) extend the same leg sideways – aiming to contract the side and back of your hip and glutes.

5. Do not to use the front of your thigh muscles to perform the side lift.

6. Do not lift too much or swing aimlessly.

Tips:

Start with small range in your lifts with a tempo of 2 counts back and 2 counts forward, or 2 counts to the side and 2 counts back in.

Begin **without** the tube, unless you have been weight training for more than a year.

Regression:

The same "side lift" may be performed lying on your side on the floor. Make sure you support your head.

Caution!

You may continue with this exercise in **T2** but ***do not use the tube***, as this may place a lot of pressure on the sacroiliac joint, which is in your tailbone/pelvis region.

TABLE 15: MOBILITY AND STABILITY DURING PREGNANCY

EXERCISE	T1 (wk1-13)	T2 (wk14-26)	T3 (wk27-40)	Absolute Beginner	Beginner	Inter-mediate	Athlete	Heart Rate	Exertion Rate
#G1 Lateral Pelvic Tilt	✓	✓	✓	✓	✓	✓	✓	Low	Low
#G2 Anterior & Posterior Pelvic Tilt	✓	✓	✓	✓	✓	✓	✓	Low	Low
#G3 Lateral Pelvic Tilt – Kneeling	✓	✓	✓	✓	✓	✓	✓	Low	Low
#G4 Russian Twist	✓	✓	No	No	✓	✓	✓	Low	Low
#G5 Muscle Energy Release	✓	✓	✓	No	✓	✓	✓	Low	Low
#G6 Hip Extension – Swiss Ball	✓	✓	No	No	✓	✓	✓	Low	Low
#G7 Hip Extension – Floor	✓	✓	No	No	✓	✓	✓	Low	Low
#G8 Hip Extension – Towel	✓	✓	✓	✓	✓	✓	✓	Low	Low
#G9 Buttock Squeeze -Tube	✓	✓	No	No	✓	✓	✓	Low	Low

Exercise H

Strengthening Exercises During Pregnancy

I cannot overemphasise the importance of strengthening your body during your pregnancy – no matter what stage you are in. This is why I have dedicated a complete chapter to help you to achieve this.

Unfortunately our brain can think, "pregnant and lifting weights – No thanks!" We tend to think that strengthening with weights means hard-core weight training at the gym, but this is not the case.

In this chapter you will find some of the most basic exercises to assist you and your body to gain strength, particularly in the areas that need it most.

It's vital that your pelvic floor muscles are strong. There is a lot of focus on strengthening your mid-section in this chapter. I start you off with the most basic "breathing 4-point kneeling" exercises and progress through to a more challenging "4-point kneeling with opposite arm and opposite leg lift". I really want you to embrace these exercises; you will love the feeling of your tummy muscles working. While your 'baby bump' is growing, it's hard to see the strength internally, but after your baby is born, your abdominals will return to shape faster. So do not get slack with yourself – do them every day if you want to – it will not hurt you, in fact it will do you and baby a world of good!

T1

For your first trimester, you may not feel like doing very much due to "morning sickness" (which can be all day – not just the morning!). For those of you who have managed to avoid this inconvenient addition to pregnancy, you can pretty much carry on your training regime, keeping your heart rate at the recommended level. Keep your heart rate below or at approximately 140 bpm to be kind to your baby because he or she is developing all their organs between weeks 8 to 13.

T2

Your second trimester is the best time to mix your training. I have always encouraged my pregnant mums to "go for it!" in the second trimester. It's that awesome time where you are not very big or uncomfortable; you generally feel great and are still having reasonable sleep. So strengthening your body during this trimester is the best choice you can make.

Any strength exercise is going to benefit you, even if you do one set of squats or push-ups on your knees or 1 abdominal exercise a day. But don't get lazy!

T3

By the time your third trimester arrives, you'll need to focus on leg strength to assist you to safely carry the increasing load of your baby and also working on your back. I have some great exercises to help keep good posture and prevent slouching. Although this may seem very basic, do make the time for these exercises as they will make your life a lot easier and less expensive with physiotherapists and massages – remember the well-proven saying, "an ounce of prevention is worth a pound of cure."

A few things to bear in mind when you are working through the exercises in this chapter:

- If I have suggested 2 sets and you are only able to do 1 set, that's fine – work progressively and do the extra set as you become stronger.
- The tempo in these exercises is very important. Remember: muscle gets stronger as it has tension going through it while stretching it.

An example of this is *Dumbbell Chest Press on the ball*, (exercise #H12) where the tempo is 3:1:2. As you lower the weight for 3 counts, the chest muscle stretches with the load of the dumbbells. Pausing for one moment creates extra tension. As you push the weight up for 2 counts, you will contract into the chest. Repeating this process will strengthen the muscle as well as create stability and good form.

Tube exercises

I have used a tube with some of the exercises for the upper body. This tube has a handle on each end, and can be used in a gym or home workout.

You can purchase a tube from a sports store or local department store. Resistance of the tube should be medium for strength work. If you are a beginner, you should start with a beginner or light tube.

Blood Pressure Cuff exercises

I use a blood pressure cuff as a bio-feedback tool to see how weak or strong core muscles are. It measures the "intra-abdominal pressure" of the core muscles (pelvic floor, transverse abdominals, and multifidus). The meter has a reading from 0 mmHg to 300mmHg. It is attached to an inflatable bag which you fold and place under your lower back – directly under your bellybutton. It can also be used in a prone (lying on tummy) position or for neck strengthening exercises but this is not appropriate during pregnancy. For our purposes, we will be using it only under the lower back for core activation and strengthening.

#H1

BRIDGE ON THE SWISS BALL – HIP EXTENSION FEET ON THE FLOOR

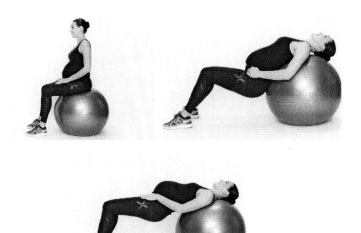

Muscles targeted: Lower back, gluteus, hips and core.

Trimester: 1, 2 and 3 if comfortable

Sets: 2-3 **Reps:** 10 **Tempo:** 3:1:2 **Rest:** 60 seconds

You may be familiar with this exercise from the "Before Pregnancy" section, as well as the "Stability" section. This exercise can be used for strengthening and stability at the same time, which is why I have included it here again.

1. Seated on the ball, walk forward and slowly lie on the ball with your head and shoulders supported. Place your hands at hip level. Bend your knees at 90 degrees directly under your feet.

2. Contract your pelvic floor muscles. Lower your hips down to a comfortable position for a count of 3, hold for 1 count and lift up in 2 counts. Feel the hips opening up in this bridge position.

3. Keep your head and shoulders on the ball and try not to move the ball in forward and backward motion. Movement should come from the hips only.

4. If this seems a little difficult, please refer to the floor version (exercise #H8). Trainers and physiotherapists refer to this as the "bridging" exercise.

5. In the later stage of your pregnancy, you should use a larger ball so that your upper body will be on an incline, and therefore the baby will not be pressing on the hip artery (inferior vena cava) and blood flow will not be restricted. This will also help with mobilising the hips, strengthening the glutes and legs without putting pressure on back, neck and shoulders.

Tip:

Before you begin coming back, gently squeeze your glutes and push through your heels for a count of 2. This can be done as a warm up before your training session or as part of your resistance program.

Regression:

If your head and shoulders are coming off the ball and your neck feels squashed, regress to the floor version.

#H2

4-Point Kneeling – Abdominal Exercise

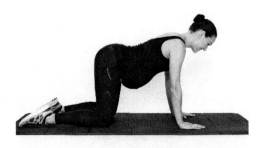

Breathing only

Muscles targeted: Internal core muscles, lower back, gluteus and hips.

Trimester: 1, 2 and 3

Sets: 2-3 **Reps:** 10 **Tempo:** Very controlled **Rest:** 60 seconds

If you are a BEGINNER, and have never done any abdominal exercis-ers, this is one of the best exercises you can do for stability, core strength and co-ordination. You need to stay focused and controlled while you perform this exercise.

1. Position yourself on all fours.

2. Ensure your hands are placed directly under the shoulders, and your knees are directly under the hips.

3. You should have two curvatures in your spine: The first is the curve of your neck, ensuring you are facing and looking at the floor. The second is your lower back, ensuring that your lower back maintains natural curve and does not go flat.

318

4. Before you start with any movement or contraction, keep in mind that your pelvis must be stable and not moving (i.e. pelvic tilting).

5. Breathe in from your diaphragm and allow your tummy to expand towards the floor. As you breathe out, **gently** lift your pelvic floor muscles internally, holding the contraction for 10 seconds. Repeat this for 10 repetitions.

6. Rest for 60 seconds and repeat for 2-3 sets.

7. Your hips or lower back **should not be flattening out at all**. Lower back should remain consistently curved.

Tip:

Your pelvic floor contractions should be 10% of what you can lift maximally. Do not overdo it as this will result in pelvic floor muscle "burn out". In the long term, this can lead to a prolapsed uterus.

#H2 - #H5 are a series of exercises that progress in degree of difficulty. If you are not familiar or comfortable with any level, I recommend that you regress as needed using the following progression, working up to #H5:

- Leg Lift only movement (#H3)
- Arm Lift only movement (#H4)
- Opposite Arm with opposite Leg movement (#H5)

#H3

4-POINT KNEELING – ABDOMINAL EXERCISE

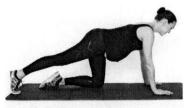 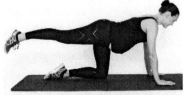

Leg only – start　　　　*Leg only – finish*

Muscles targeted: Internal core muscles, lower back, gluteus and hips.

Trimester: 1, 2 and 3

Sets: 2-3 **Reps:** 10 **Tempo:** 3:1:3 **Rest:** 60 seconds

Leg Lift only movement

1.   Before you begin, ensure your pelvic floor muscles are activated.

2.   Lift up your extended leg in a controlled lift for 3 counts, hold for 1 count, and 3 counts down. Repeat 10 times.

3.   Your leg should be very straight. Do not bend your knee, and only go to your hip-height.

4.   Repeat with the other leg.

5.   You should notice your glutes working and your deep core muscles will be working constantly through each lift.

Tip:

If you feel you have lost your pelvic floor contraction during the lift, re-group and start again.

#H4

4–POINT KNEELING – ABDOMINAL EXERCISE

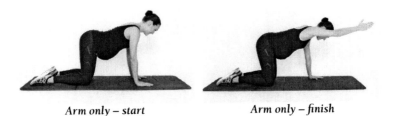

Arm only – start   *Arm only – finish*

Muscles targeted: Internal core muscles, lower back, gluteus and hips.

Trimester: 1, 2 and 3

Sets: 1-2 **Reps:** 10 **Tempo:** 3:1:3 **Rest:** 60 seconds

One Arm Lift only movement

Carrying out the one arm lift on its own will help you be aware of your shoulder stabilisation. You may only need to do this few times before you can progress to opposite arm and leg movement.

1. As with the leg lift, lift one arm completing 10 repetitions on each arm. Repeat on the other side.

2. Focus on the pelvic floor muscles also, as this will be pre-programming the muscles for the next progression.

3. When you feel you are competent with your posture and strength, you can progress on to the alternate arm and leg lift.

#H5

4-POINT KNEELING – ABDOMINAL EXERCISE

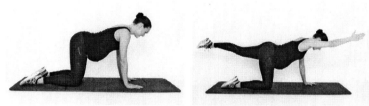

Opposite arm with opposite leg movement

Muscles targeted: Internal core muscles, lower back, gluteus and hips.

Trimester: 1, 2 and 3

Sets: 2-3 **Reps:** 10 **Tempo:** 3:1:3 **Rest:** 60 seconds

1. Begin on all fours. Take a breath in from the diaphragm and as you breathe out start lifting your pelvic floor muscles only (the bellybutton will do what it should, subconsciously).

2. After you are holding the contraction, you can lift the opposite arm and leg off the floor.

3. Maintain your contraction throughout the whole movement, while **simultaneously** lifting your opposite arm and leg. This is where you will need to pay special attention, so that arm and leg extend without your body moving at all.

4. Hold extended position for 1 count and very, very slowly return the arm and leg simultaneously to the starting position.

5. If your leg or arm land back on the floor at separate times from each other, then you will need to work on the tempo and quality of your movement.

6. Be careful to slow things down; do not rush your midsection contractions for the sake of 10 repetitions. You may only manage 5 repetitions to begin with, which is fine.

#H6

LEG CURLS – SWISS BALL

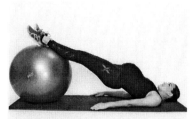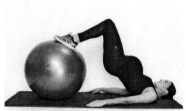

Muscles targeted: Hamstrings, gluteus and core.

Trimester: 1 and 2 (only if comfortable)

Sets: 2-3 **Reps:** 10 **Tempo:** 3:1:3 **Rest:** 60 seconds

During T2, you will need to assess your ability to do this exercise. It may be fine at the beginning if you have been doing these during pre-pregnancy and in T1. However as your baby grows, you may not feel comfortable or confident and if this is the case, I recommend you do not do this exercise.

1. Lie on your back with your heels and calves on top of the ball.

2. Ensure you have equal space between both legs, and that your feet are in the middle of the ball, so you don't roll off side. Place your palms down and out to 45 degrees for support.

3. Contract your pelvic floor muscles first. While maintaining the contraction, lift your hips up and stabilise. With controlled form, bring the ball close to your hamstrings and glutes – thus performing a hamstring curl.

4. Maintaining the pelvis alignment, slowly return to the start position.

5. Keep your toes pointed, as this should make it easier to maintain your balance.

Regression:

If you are not able to perform the leg curl, go back to the hip extension alone. Place your calves on the ball, with straight legs – lift your hips off the floor and lower your hips to the starting position. Repeat 10 times.

#H7

SWISS BALL WALL SQUAT

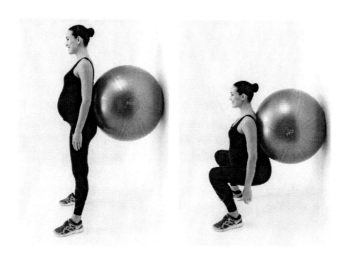

Muscles targeted: Thighs, gluteus and core.

Trimester: 1, 2 and 3

Sets: 3 **Reps:** 10-20 **Tempo:** 3:1:3 **Rest:** 60 seconds

Using a Swiss ball is a very effective and safe way to learn how to squat during pregnancy. Make sure you have a safe wall to use. When performing a squat it is important to have your pelvic floor muscles and multifidus working together to prevent lower back problems.

1. Against a wall, place the Swiss ball in the small of your back, and comfortably lean on the ball. Take your feet slightly forward with feet hip-width apart.

2. Draw your pelvic floor muscles up and the lower portion of your abdomen in. Now you are ready to squat. Do not do squats without your pelvic floor muscles contracting. (Your mutifidus only

contracts when you activate your pelvic floor, which also protects your back.) Aim to comfortably do 10-15 repetitions if you are a beginner. If you are used to squatting, increase up to 25 repetitions.

3. Depth of the squat should not exceed the 90 degrees at the knees, as you will lose your pelvic floor and lower abdominal contraction. On your way up, push through your heels and be aware of the glutes working to help you to lift yourself.

Tips:

Your strength, flexibility and stamina will determine how many repetitions you are capable of performing. Sets will depend on how much time you have as well as your level of fitness. Tempo can change to 3:1:2, going down for 3 counts, holding for 1 and coming up in 2. Or going down for 4 counts, holding for 1 count and coming up in 3. You may need to watch this, as you are better off doing the slow tempo, so that you don't lose the pelvic floor contraction through the lowering and lifting stage.

The depth of your squat should only be as low as you are comfortable. Keep the glutes and hips against the ball the whole time.

Caution!

If you experience any knee pain, please seek medical advice.

#H8

SWISS BALL WALL SQUAT WITH MEDICINE BALL

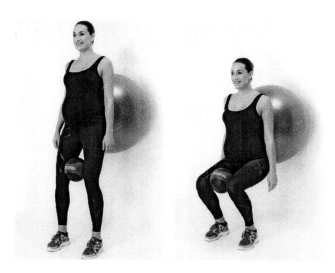

Muscles targeted: Inner thighs, front and back of thighs, gluteus and core.

Trimester: 1 and 2

Sets: 3 **Reps:** 12 **Tempo:** 3:1:3 **Rest:** 60 seconds

Provided there are no pelvic floor or pubic symphysis issues, this exercise can be effective in getting inner thighs involved.

This exercise works extremely well when combined with some hip strengthening exercises. Stretching the inner thigh in the beginning of the workout will really benefit this squat.

This is a variation of the squat and not to be performed in addition to the regular squat.

1. Following from the ball wall-squat position, place the small 1 or 2 kg medicine ball (or a rolled up large towel) in between your thighs. You may need your feet closer than hip-width apart in order to hold the ball. Draw your pelvic floor muscles up and the lower portion of your abdomen in before you start to go down in your squat.

2. As you begin to squat, gently squeeze the medicine ball between your thighs. Keep this squeeze until you have returned to the top.

3. Go down for 3 counts, hold for 1 and come up for 3 counts. This will ensure a correct pelvic floor contraction.

Tip:

Stretch your inner-thigh while seated on the ball after each set. See stretch #F4 – Swiss ball version.

#H9

SIDE-ON – BALL WALL SQUAT

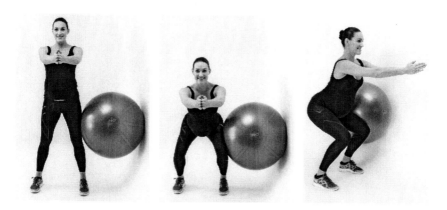

Muscles targeted: Thighs, gluteus, hips and core.

Trimester: 1, 2 and 3

Sets: 2-3 **Reps:** 10 **Tempo:** 3:1:2 **Rest:** 60 seconds

In the past, I have had some clients with various knee issues, which resulted in their hips also being affected. This particular squat places emphasis on strengthening some of the weak hip muscles. If you have any issues with your knees or hips, please check with your health care practitioner and get clearance to do this particular exercise.

1. Position yourself sideways with the ball on the outside of your thigh just above the knee level. Take a diaphragmatic breath in and as you breathe out, lift your pelvic floor up and draw your lower abdomen (or bellybutton) inwards towards your spine.

2. Go down for a count of 3, hold the position for 1 and come up for a count of 2. During your squat position, gently push with the knee onto the ball.

3. Do as many as you are comfortable, maintaining good hip alignment and curvature in your lower back.

Tip:

Holding your arms out in front of you can help you to stabilise and perform the squat with better posture.

Regression:

Partial Squat – only go down as far as comfortable.

Caution!

If you notice any knee, hip or back soreness, stop immediately and seek medical advice.

#H10

ROTATIONAL LUNGE WITH A MEDICINE BALL

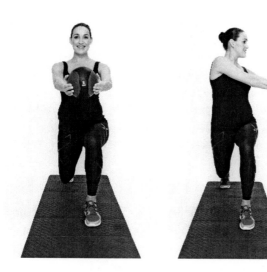

Muscles targeted: Whole body.

Trimester: 1 only, and only if accustomed to this exercise before falling pregnant

Sets: 2 **Reps:** 8-12 **Tempo:** 2:0:2 **Rest:** 30 seconds

Once you have mastered the lunge, either on the ball on the wall or free-standing, your next progression involves some rotational movement. Rotational movement is involved in a mother's everyday routine: going grocery shopping, picking up bags or laundry, twisting with loading and offloading shopping bags or prams from your car and so on. Building strength in this area will increase your stamina and lessen the chance of injury. This is an excellent exercise as it involves the oblique muscles (waist muscles) which together work with your transverse abdominals (core).

1. Taking a medicine ball, begin with a split stance. Ensure your back foot is loaded on your toes, and your body weight is distributed evenly between the front and back leg.

2. Before you start your rotational lunge, connect your pelvic floor and deep abdominal muscles in. As you lunge down, rotate to the outside of your front leg and keep your eyes fixed on the medicine ball.

3. Relax your shoulders and arms. All your movement should be coming from your legs, glutes and your midsection.

4. Attempt 10-20 repetitions with good form, resting for 30-60 seconds between each set. You can stay in the lunge position, or come up with each rep and lunge down while rotating. Always breathe out as you come up. You can add another set, or if you are feeling strong, increase the repetitions to 20 on each side.

Tips:

Your medicine ball can vary from 1kg-5kg, again depending on your training age and level of strength and fitness. Make sure you choose the appropriate ball weight for your level.

This exercise can also be performed with a cable machine at the same tempo, however make sure you stay in control as your core muscles must control the pull and release of the weight.

#H11

Rotational Lunge and Extension With Medicine Ball

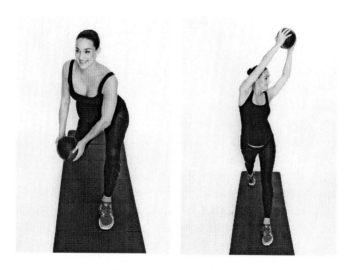

Muscles targeted: Whole body.

Trimester: 1 only and only if accustomed to this exercise before falling pregnant

Sets: 2 **Reps:** 8-20 **Tempo:** 2:0:2 **Rest:** 30 seconds

This exercise is the progression of the previous exercise, with an extension of arms towards the ceiling. Picking up washing and putting it on the line would be the constant domestic practice you will become well-acquainted with.

1. Begin with a split stance. Ensure your back foot is loaded on your toes and your body weight is distributed evenly between the front and back leg.

2. Connect your pelvic floor and deep abdominal muscles in before you begin your lunge. Rotate and flex (bend forward and down) on the inside of your front leg. Keep your eyes fixed on the medicine ball.

3. Relax your shoulders and arms. All your movement should be coming from your legs, glutes and midsection.

4. Using your glutes by pushing through your front heel, lift the ball up towards the ceiling with both arms straight, and **DO NOT** lock the elbows.

5. Extend and feel the lengthening of your torso.

6. Repeat on the other side.

7. If you are a **beginner**, start with 8 repetitions and go down for 2 counts without resting at the bottom; come up fast for 2 counts.

8. If you do lunges regularly, then really focus on the extension of your torso. Ensure that you are not overstretching. Perhaps visualise this exercise as if you are putting washing on the clothes line. You can increase the repetitions to 20 to build your strength for domestic chores!

9. Always breathe out as you come up.

Tip:

Your medicine-ball can vary from 1kg-2kg depending on your training age and level of strength and fitness. Do not use anything heavier, as this may cause your lower back to hyper-extend (excessive arch in the lower back) and cause possible injury.

#H12

CHEST PRESS ON SWISS BALL WITH DUMBBELLS

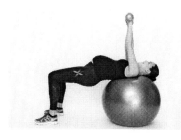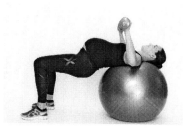

Muscles targeted: Chest, triceps, legs, gluteus and core.

Trimester: 1, 2 and 3

Sets: 3 **Reps:** 15-20 **Tempo:** 3:1:2 **Rest:** 60 seconds

This is a favourite of my pregnant clients. It works your chest while also working your glutes. It also creates greater stability throughout the midsection.

1. From a seated position, walk forward with your feet and lie back on the Swiss ball with your head and shoulders well supported. Knees are in line with the heels.

2. Ensure both arms are straight with "soft" elbows (do not lock them out) and are positioned above your chest, not your face.

3. Lower your arms for 3 counts and hold for 1 count. Press evenly with both arms in 2 counts, returning arms above your chest to your starting position.

4. As you are opening with your arms, feel the chest stretch and your shoulder blades moving towards the ball, as you slowly lower both arms until the elbows are at 90 degrees.

Tip:

In T3, lower your hips down to the floor slightly, so that the pressure is not on your back, and also not restricting blood flow. Or you can use a larger ball and position yourself in an incline position.

#H13

SINGLE ARM TUBE ROW

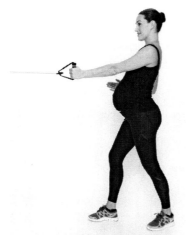 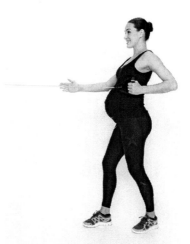

Right leg forward, left leg back,
grasp handle with left hand

Pull handle with left hand, while
extending right hand in front

Muscles targeted: Arms (biceps), upper back and core.

Trimester: 1, 2 and 3

Sets: 3 **Reps:** 10-15 **Tempo:** 2:1:3 **Rest:** 30-60 seconds

This is a back strengthening exercise that involves rotation during a single arm pull. You will need a rubber tube with individual handles and a solid object to wrap the tube around, so that it is stable and stays fixed as you perform the exercise.

1. Your stance is opposite arm to the opposite leg. The photographs show right leg forward and left leg back. It may be more comfortable to have your back heel off the floor and up on your toes. Contract your pelvic and deep abdominal muscles.

2. Hold the handle of the tube with your left hand as in a hand-shake position.

3. Your opposite arm (right) will begin bending at the waist as you are performing your row with your left arm. Then, your right arm will be moving forward into an extension acting as a lever, while the left arm is performing another row. Ensure your head, shoulders and hips are in line, and that your hips are not twisting.

4. Breathe in; as you breathe out, pull with your right arm until you feel the back shoulder blade squeezing. Pull for a count of 2, hold for 1 and release for 3 counts.

5. Complete 10 to 15 repetitions on one arm and change to the other side.

6. Rest for 30-60 seconds and repeat for 3 sets.

#H14

STANDING TUBE ROW

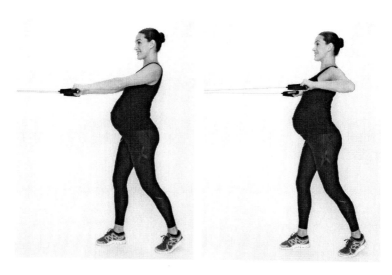

Muscles targeted: Core, upper back, biceps and shoulders.

Trimester: 1, 2 and 3

Sets: 3 **Reps:** 10-15 **Tempo:** 2:1:3 **Rest:** 60 seconds

This is another back strengthening exercise. Notice in the photograph the model has both elbows out and away from the body. This exercise is performed standing with the elbows travelling outwards.

The exercise that follows this one, (seated row on the ball – exercise #H15), is performed with both elbows tucked in at the waist while pulling.

1. Position yourself far enough from your pole (or support object), so that you have some resistance in the tube.

2. Take a split stance distributing your bodyweight evenly on both legs (see exercise #H13).

3. Maintain the curvature in your lower back and neck. Do not poke your head forward during this exercise.

4. Breathe in; as you breathe out pull the tube evenly with both arms, palms facing the floor. Pull for 2 counts, hold for 1 and while still maintaining contraction in your mid back, release the tube slowly for a count of 3.

5. Complete 10-15 repetitions with 3 sets.

6. Rest between each set for 60 seconds.

Tip:

Concentrate on the shoulder blades coming towards the spine and feel the middle of the back get strong.

#H15

SEATED ROW ON SWISS BALL WITH TUBE

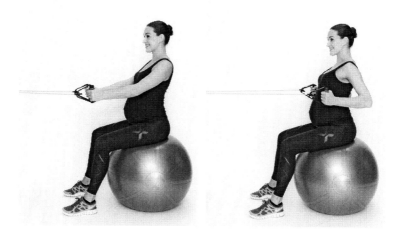

Muscles targeted: Core, upper back, biceps and shoulders.

Trimester: 1, 2 and 3

Sets: 3 **Reps:** 10-15 **Tempo:** 2:1:3 **Rest:** 60 seconds

This is one of my favourite exercises for the back, as it is very effective for back strengthening. You will likely spend many hours feeding (breast or bottle) and your upper back will start to stretch and feel weak. For this reason you need to strengthen this area as much as possible and keep it strong.

1. Sit on the Swiss ball with a tall posture, placing your arms in front of your tummy. Keep your legs fairly close to the ball with knees bent at 90 degrees.

2. Hold the handles in a "thumbs up" position.

3. Pay particular attention to your upper body alignment, keeping it lengthened. Make sure you have your shoulders down and shoulder blades slightly drawn towards your spine.

4. Breathe in; as you breathe out pull the tube for 2 counts. Focus on your elbows squeezing the upper back for 1 count. Release for 3 counts and repeat for 10-15 repetitions.

5. Rest for 60 seconds between each set.

#H16

DUMBBELL BICEP CURLS – SEATED ON THE SWISS BALL WITH ONE LEG UP

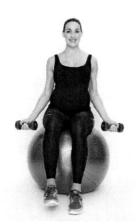 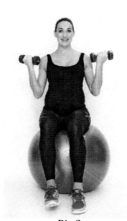 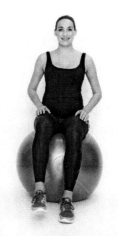

Pic 1
Start with hands at thigh level with palms facing up.

Pic 2
Curl up to shoulder height

Pic 3
See tips.

Muscles targeted: Core and biceps.

Trimester: 1, 2 and 3

Sets: 2 **Reps:** 12 on each leg **Tempo:** 3:1:3 **Rest:** 60 seconds

The Swiss ball will always be an unstable environment while you are training. Taking 1 leg off the floor while performing an upper body movement, will call on the deep abdominal wall for stabilisation, which is again great for core stability and strength. However, if you have only just started using the ball, it would be wise to begin with both feet grounded.

1. Contract your deep abdominal wall and lift the pelvic floor muscles up and away from the Swiss ball. Sit tall with good posture in your upper back.

2. Lift 1 leg off the floor.

3. Starting with hands at thigh level with palms facing up, curl up for 3 counts, hold for 1 count and lower for 3 counts.

4. Complete 12 repetitions with the arms and then change legs. Rest 60 seconds and repeat for 2 sets.

Tips:

Firstly, practice lifting 1 leg off the floor. Hold each lift for 10 seconds and repeat on the other side. Keep doing this until you feel you have done enough, by doing this you will prepare your core muscles to progress to adding an arm line.

Dumbbells are optional. Choose light weights (1-3kg).

If you have not done this exercise before pregnancy, do not use the dumbbell until you are confident and strong enough in your core muscles.

#H17

LATERAL DUMBBELL RAISES – SEATED ON SWISS BALL

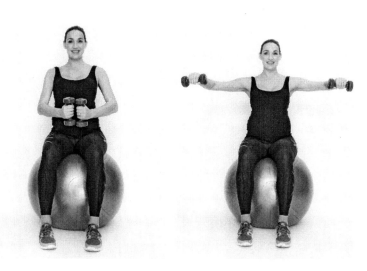

Muscles targeted: Core and shoulders.

Trimester: 1, 2 and 3

Sets: 2-3 **Reps:** 10-20 **Tempo:** 2:1:3 **Rest:** 60 seconds

1. Contract your deep abdominal muscles and lift the pelvic floor up and away from the Swiss ball.

2. Hold your dumbbells in each hand as if you are holding 2 glasses of water. Position them in front of your bellybutton.

3. Breathe in; as you breathe out lift both arms for 2 counts. Both elbows need to be at 90 degrees or like two L shapes. Hold for 1 count. Keeping your posture tall, return to your start position in 3 counts.

4. Perform this exercise for 2 to 3 sets, with 10-20 repetitions and lightweights of 1-2 kg.

Tips:

Lifting 1 leg off the floor during this exercise is an option.

If you have trained for stability before falling pregnant, you can use 2-3kg dumbbells.

#H18

DUMBBELL SHOULDER PRESS – SEATED ON SWISS BALL

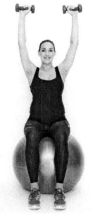
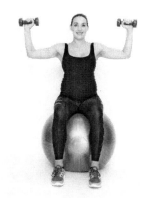

Pic 1
Start with dumbbells above your shoulders

Pic 2
Lower arms until elbows are shoulder height

Muscles targeted: Core muscles and shoulders.

Trimester: 1 and 2

Sets: 2 **Reps:** 10-15 **Tempo:** 3:1:2 **Rest:** 60 seconds

1. Seated on the Swiss ball, contract your deep abdominal muscles and lift the pelvic floor muscles up and away from the ball.

2. Lift both arms up above the shoulders without locking your elbows. This is your starting position as shown in pic 1.

3. With a normal breathing pattern, start by lowering both arms until elbows are at shoulder height for 3 counts, hold for 1 and lift for 2 counts.

4. Complete 2 sets of 10-15 repetitions, with 60 seconds rest.

Tip:

If you have been training with good core stability, then you may wish to attempt lifting one leg off the floor. *I do not recommend you attempt this without prior training to this level.*

Caution!

If you have high blood pressure or shoulder issues do not perform this exercise.

#H19

DEEP ABDOMINAL WALL – CORE STRENGTH WITH BLOOD PRESSURE CUFF

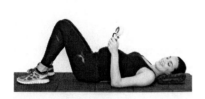 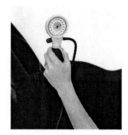

This is one of the best and most effective exercises to strengthen pelvic floor and reduce hip instability.

If you do not have a blood pressure cuff, you can purchase one from your chemist, drug store or medical supplier for about $50.

Muscles targeted: Pelvic floor, transverse abdominals and obliques (core).

Trimester: 1 and 2

Sets: 2 Reps: 10 **Hold:** 10 second **Rest:** 60-90 seconds

1. Lie on your back with both knees bent and hip-width apart.

2. Place the folded deflated cuff in the lumbar area (lower back) directly underneath your bellybutton region, and ensure it is evenly distributed on both sides.

3. Make sure your lower back is relaxed and has its own natural curve – neutral position. Do not arch your lower back to create room for the cuff.

4. Ensure you have even pressure on both sides of your lower back. If not, adjust the cuff from side to side, so that it is symmetrical and placed in the centre of your lower back.

5. Pump up the cuff until the needle goes to 40mmHg. During this time, maintain the position of your lower back. This is going to be the base for your contraction. Do not arch your back.

6. Breathe in diaphragmatically. Your diaphragm sits between your ribcage and bellybutton. (Ensure that your lungs are not expanding, as it's the diaphragm that should be expanding first).

7. As you breathe out, slowly and gently lift your pelvic floor muscles in. Your pelvic floor muscle is internal – however it extends to your anal passage – so ensure that you are contracting this area also. It should be a very gentle lift, and not a sharp pull or a strong contraction. This part is the internal lift of your pelvic floor.

8. While maintaining the lift of your pelvic floor muscles, you will need to draw the lower portion of your abdomen inwards (or towards the spine). At the same time, gently press your lower back down on the pressure of the cuff.

9. This will create pressure in your deep abdominal wall which the needle should measure as 50-60mmHg. Hold this pressure or contraction for 10 seconds and relax for 10 seconds. Repeat for 10 repetitions. All movements should be very slow and controlled.

10. After each set, roll on to your left side and recover for 60-90 seconds. Continue this for 2-3 sets and only do as much as you can.

11. A description for "intensity" would be at about 10-20% of what you are able to do at your maximum effort. It's going to feel very gentle, as if you are not doing very much.

12. Don't cheat yourself by thinking you should be doing more. Doing 10 repetitions with 10 second contractions will get the muscles working quite quickly.

Tips:

When I was pregnant and suffering with sciatica, my physiotherapist gave me a similar exercise but pressing on my hand under my lower back for 10 seconds. I went home and did my committed exercise; however I thought I had to squash my hand with my lower back in order to get a good contraction. This is not the case.

While this exercise may still be prescribed, the blood pressure cuff is a visual tool for proper contraction and activation of the "intra-abdominal" pressure without over-activating. Remember that over-contracting these muscles may cause prolapsed uterus in the long term.

TABLE 16: STRENGTHENING EXERCISES DURING PREGNANCY

EXERCISE	T1 (wk1-13)	T2 (wk14-26)	T3 (wk27-40)	Absolute Beginner	Beginner	Inter-mediate	Athlete	Heart Rate	Exertion Rate
#H1 Bridge on the Swiss Ball	✓	✓	✓	No	✓	✓	✓	Low	Low
#H2 4-Point Kneeling	✓	✓	✓	✓	✓	✓	✓	Low	Low
#H3 4-Point Kneeling – Leg	✓	✓	✓	✓	✓	✓	✓	Low	Low
#H4 4-Point Kneeling – Arm	✓	✓	✓	✓	✓	✓	✓	Low	Low
#H5 4-Point Kneeling – Arm and Leg	✓	✓	✓	No *	No *	✓	✓	Low	Low
#H6 Leg Curls - Swiss Ball	✓	✓	No	No	✓	✓	✓	Low	Medium
#H7 Swiss Ball Wall Squat	✓	✓	✓	✓	✓	✓	✓	Low	Medium
#H8 Ball Squats – Med Ball	✓	✓	No	No	✓	✓	✓	Low	Medium
#H9 Side-on - Ball Wall Squats	✓	✓	No	No	No	✓	✓	Low	Medium
#H10 Rotational Lunge – Med ball	✓	No	No	No	✓**	✓	✓	Low	Medium
#H11 Rotational Lunge and Extension	✓	***	No	No	No	✓	✓	Low	Medium/High
#H12 Chest Press – Swiss Ball	✓	✓	✓	✓	✓	✓	✓	Low	Medium
#H13 Single Arm Row	✓	✓	✓	✓	✓	✓	✓	Low	Low
#H14 Standing Tube Row	✓	✓	✓	✓	✓	✓	✓	Low	Medium
#H15 Seated Row – Swiss ball	✓	✓	✓	✓	✓	✓	✓	Low	Low
#H16 DB Bicep Curl	✓	✓	✓	No	No	✓	✓	Low	Low
#H17 Lateral Raises on Swiss Ball	✓	✓	✓	No	No	✓	✓	Low	Low
#H18 DB Shoulder Press	✓	✓	No	No	✓	✓	✓	Low	Low
#H19 Blood Pressure Cuff	✓	✓	✓	✓	✓	✓	✓	Low	Low

* An absolute beginner is best to practice 4-point kneeling with breathing and contracting the pelvic floor effectively before moving on to arms and legs being extended.

** Rotational Lunge with medicine ball for beginners is OK, however you will need to concentrate on technique and make sure your knees are not buckling inwards as you go down into your lunge.

*** Rotational Lunge with Overhead Extension for T2, read your body. Do not over extend with the arms overhead. The idea is to use your arms as in functional movement e.g. putting washing on the line. If you are able to continue, do this for as long as you are able within comfort. But as you get bigger and it's no longer comfortable, then do not continue with the overhead – just do a partial lunge, which goes down only half-way. Again, you may only be able to do these half-way through T2. Your body will tell you how much you can do. Be sensible, and take care of yourself.

Dangerous Exercises for Post-Natal Women

As I mentioned in Chapter 7 "Your Fitness Program After Pregnancy", many women are extremely keen to get their pre-baby shape back. Often they will join a gym and attack exercises such as crunches in an attempt to get back their flat tummy. I do not recommend this approach. Even though you may see many people doing these kinds of exercises, this does not mean that they are the best or safest exercise for you.

Follow the advice of your doctor, see a physiotherapist or chiropractor and get your body back in alignment, so that you don't injure yourself and your exercise is enjoyable. We all love results - doing things that are safe and effective that produces these results, means that we will stay with the program.

The following are some of the dangerous exercises for post-delivery. Women who choose to do these exercises may believe they are benefitting, but in reality, they do much more harm than good **so please stay away from these**. You will notice I offer some safe and effective alternatives to each of the dangerous exercises.

CRUNCHES WITH FEET LOCKED

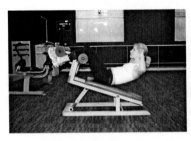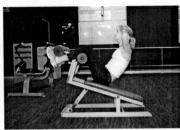

In my experience with this particular version of the crunch, the hip flexor muscle (psoas), which is already short and tight, becomes even tighter during the crunch.

When the psoas gets tight then one of the lower back muscles (quadratus lumborum) gets tight also – it's a recipe for injury and lower back problems.

These two muscles are overactive with daily activities and there is absolutely no need to train them to become even tighter. If anything, the crunch should be reversed to open up the hips and torso.

If you are after a "two-pack" this is the way to achieve it. However if you want balance between abdominals and a strong lower back then this is not the exercise for you in the early stages of post-delivery.

A safer alternative is #D28 *Crunches on Swiss Ball*.

Lower Abdominals – Leg Raises

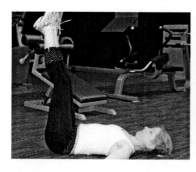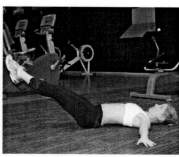

Much of what I described about the crunch with feet locked also applies to this exercise. I see many women end up with a sore back after doing this.

Some women have a heavier lower body than upper body. The load going through the lower back as you are desperately trying to engage the lower abdominals is enormous!

You may have seen women trying to do this and their lower back is arching as their legs go down.

It's a great exercise, however more suited to intermediate/advanced training – not post-natal. I do not include this exercise for anyone until they have progressed gradually with good balance between lower back and deep abdominal work.

One way of self-assessing is by doing a full hover or bridge for 1 minute and progressing to 2 minutes without arching the back, and then you should be able to perform this exercise.

A great alternative is #H5 *4-Point Kneeling – abdominal exercise*, which is fantastic post-pregnancy. When you are stronger in your deep abdominals (core), then you can go to #D24 *Prone Jack Knife* (tummy tuck).

LOWER ABDOMINALS – LEG RAISES WITH SWISS BALL

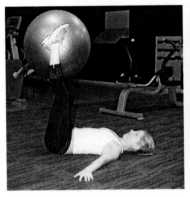 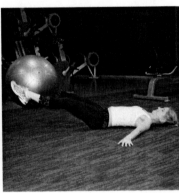

This is the same exercise as the previous, except adding the ball makes it a bit more challenging. The added tension is in the inner thigh holding the large ball, but all the other factors remain the same.

This is a very popular exercise in many gyms, but please prevent any lower back pain by eliminating advanced exercises such as these in the early stages of post-delivery.

A great alternative is #H5 *4-Point Kneeling – abdominal exercise*, which is fantastic post-pregnancy. When you are stronger in your deep abdominals (core), then you can go to #D24 *Prone Jack Knife* (tummy tuck).

Deadlift with a Bar

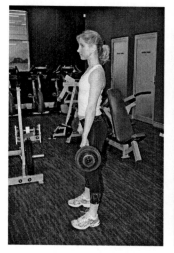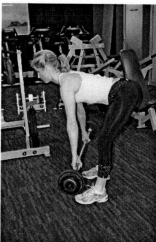

One of the much-loved hamstring exercises in the gym is the deadlift. You will see many women do this exercise, as it really works the hamstrings and glutes. This is an advanced exercise, which is mostly prescribed to athletes or women who are competing for sculpting or bodybuilding competitions.

If you perform it during the post-delivery period, it can cause pain or injury to your lower back, which is why you must avoid it. Due to the hormone Relaxin, many ligaments in your pelvis have stretched past their normal range for delivery, and loading up the lower back in this way will only create problems both short term and long term.

The problem with this exercise is that if you do not have adequate core strength (pelvic floor and deep abdominals are not stabilising the spine or protecting the back), the weak lower back takes the majority of the load.

Posture during the exercise is sometimes compromised by rounding off the back, thus applying more pressure to the mid and lower back discs.

I strongly advise you not do this exercise for at least twelve months after the birth, and then only under the supervision of a qualified therapist or trainer.

A better exercise for the hamstrings is exercise #H6 *Leg Curls – Swiss Ball*. This is safe and effective.

Back Extension – with or without Weight

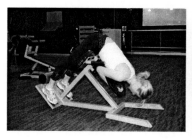 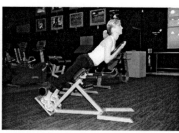

This is another exercise where the back is weak and compromised either with or without load (e.g. weighted plate). Your lower back has been continually loaded for the duration of your pregnancy, especially in T3. You need to relieve this load and strengthen the surrounding postural muscles around the torso – this is why this exercise is not good in the post-natal period.

A common mistake with performing the back extension is the neck and lower back are hyper-extended, putting pressure on the cervical and lumbar discs.

Alternative exercises that are safe and effective are #C1 *Hip Extension*, #C3 *Hip Extension – Swiss ball version* or #H5 *4-Point Kneeling – abdominal exercise.*

PROGRAM CHARTS

In this chapter I have provided programs to suit each level of experience and phase of pregnancy. Toward the end of the programs, I have included a program specifically for those with hip and knee issues, along with a glossary of self-myofascial releases, stretches and stability exercises.

You should first determine your level of experience and review the appropriate programs. Each program is designed to be a standalone workout that you can perform in a session at home or at the gym.

The exercise numbers refer to the exercise descriptions in the previous chapters. You should review the instructions for each exercise and the tips to be sure that you are doing them correctly. In some cases I have given additional instructions in the program charts to provide you with additional guidance. For example, the exercise description may give several options, but in the program for your level I recommend a particular variation.

I recommend you print the charts and refer to them during your workouts.

You should aim to do a minimum of 3 program sessions a week, depending on your fitness level and experience. As you gain fitness, you may supplement these sessions with cardiovascular exercise (e.g. a walk or run), yoga or Pilates classes, or therapeutic exercise. This will add variety to your program and accelerate your progress. Just be sure to train at your level and avoid over training.

Your training week as a beginner to intermediate could look like this:

	Week 1	Week 2	Week 3	Week 4
Monday	Program	Program	Program	Program
Tuesday	Rest day	Walk	Pilates class	Rest day
Wednesday	Program	Program	Program	Program
Thursday	Rest day	Rest day	Rest day	Yoga class
Friday	Program	Program	Program	Program
Saturday	Rest day	Walk	Walk or Run	Walk or Run
Sunday	Rest day	Rest day	Rest day	Rest day

As you progress in your fitness, you can add exercise days or increase the intensity of your workouts. However, I recommend that you do not weight-train the same muscles on consecutive days and you should have at least one rest day per week. Example would be large muscle groups like the chest, back or legs. These muscles need a day to recover.

Absolute Beginners and Beginners will notice that I have given only one program that you should do for a 6 week block before you progress. This will help you become really familiar with the exercises and allow you to follow the instructions closely to ensure that you are doing them correctly.

Over time you may become bored with doing the same programs. In that case, you should substitute some exercises or a complete program appropriate to your fitness level. But don't advance too quickly.

Make sure you are doing a variety of activities in addition to the programs. If you like the outdoors, choose activities such as walking, running, hiking, swimming at the beach, golf etc. If you prefer indoor activities, then Yoga, Pilates and Qi Qong would be calming and de-stressing.

PROGRAM 1

BEFORE PREGNANCY FOR ABSOLUTE BEGINNER

HOME WORKOUT

TRAINING AGE: 0-6 MONTHS

DURATION: 6 WEEKS

Exercise	Exercise	Sets	Reps	Tempo/Hold	Weight	Rest	Notes
	MUSCLE SPASM RELEASES – MYOFASCIAL RELEASE ON FOAM ROLLER						
#A5	Hips and ITB	1	1	15 secs		nil	
#A6	Buttocks and Piriformis	1	1	10-20 secs		nil	
#A9	Front Thigh	1	1	15 secs		nil	
	STRETCHES						
#B2	Neck – Side	1	1	10 secs		nil	
#B7	Upper Back	1	1	10 secs		nil	
#B14	Hip and Inner Thigh	1	1	60 sec		nil	choose wall or floor version
#B15	Calf	1	1	20 secs		nil	
	STABILITY						
#C1	Hip Extension – Floor	1	10	323		nil	
#C6	Basic 4 Point Kneeling	1	10	10 sec hold		nil	
#C9	Leg Lift – Swiss Ball	1	10	222		30 secs	single leg version only
#C10	Prone Cobra – Swiss Ball	1	10	222		nil	with or without the ball
	WEIGHTS						
#D1	Calf Raises	1	10	213	bodyweight	60 secs	
#D3	Swiss Ball Wall Squats	1	10	313	bodyweight	60 secs	
#D22	Seated Row	1	12	213	tube	60 secs	
#D30	Push-ups – Floor	1	10	312	bodyweight	60 secs	
#D40	DB Bicep Curls	1	12	213	2kg	60 secs	
#D42	DB Lateral Raise	1	12	213	2kg	60 secs	
#D44	Tricep Dips	1	12	312	bodyweight	60 secs	

Notes:

As you progress, add in a 20 minute walk on the alternate days. Do all your stretches and stability work and then do a walk.

This program is only for 6 weeks, so take advantage of learning how to do the stretches and stability, so that the weights will become easier. Feel free to upgrade to 3kg dumbbells.

PROGRAM 2
BEFORE PREGNANCY FOR ABSOLUTE BEGINNER
HOME WORKOUT
TRAINING AGE: 0-6 MONTHS
DURATION: 6 WEEKS – PROGRESSION FROM PROGRAM 1

Exercise	Exercise	Sets	Reps	Tempo/ Hold	Weight	Rest	Notes
	MUSCLE SPASM RELEASES – MYOFASCIAL RELEASE ON FOAM ROLLER						
#A1	Neck Release	1	1	10 secs		nil	
#A2	Latissimus Dorsi	1	1	10 secs		nil	
#A4	Lower Back	1	1	20 secs		nil	
#A5	Hips and ITB	1	1	15 secs		nil	
#A6	Buttocks and Piriformis	1	1	20 secs		nil	
#A7	Calf	1	1	15 secs		nil	
	STRETCHES						
#B14	Hip and Inner Thigh	1	1	60 secs		nil	
#B1	Neck – Back	1	1	20 secs		nil	
#B10	Lower Back	1	1	20 secs		nil	
#B11	McKenzie Press-up	1	10	323		nil	
#B13	Hip and Thigh	1	1	10 secs		nil	
	STABILITY						
#C1	Hip Extension – Floor	1	10	323		30-60 secs	
#C5	Hip Extension – Inner Thigh	1	10	222		30-60 secs	
#C6	Basic 4 Point Kneeling	1	10	10 secs		60 secs	
#C9	Leg Lift – Swiss Ball	1	10	222		nil	
#C10	Prone Cobra – Swiss Ball	1	10	222		30 sec	
CARDIO	Alternate days you will do cardiovascular exercises e.g. walk, swim or bike ride for 30 minutes.						
	WEIGHTS						
#D1	Calf Raises	1	10	213	bodyweight	30 secs	
#D3	Swiss Ball Wall Squats	1	10	313	bodyweight	30 secs	
#D6	Hip Extension – Swiss Ball	1	10	213	bodyweight	30secs	
#D9	Lunge – Swiss Ball on Wall	1	12	312	bodyweight	30 secs	
#D22	Seated Row	1	12	213	light tube	30secs	Use Swiss ball and tube
#D31	Push-ups – Wall	1	10	312	bodyweight	30secs	

Notes:

Add on cardiovascular workouts on alternate days, or choose a therapeutic exercise such as Qi Qong, or Feldenkrais or Yoga.

This program is only for 6 weeks, so take advantage of learning how to do the stretches and stability, so that the weights become easier. Increase the repetitions from 10 to 20 as you become stronger.

PROGRAM 3
BEFORE PREGNANCY FOR BEGINNER
GYM WORKOUT
TRAINING AGE: 0-6 MONTHS
DURATION: 6 WEEKS

Exercise	Exercise	Sets	Reps	Tempo/Hold	Weight	Rest	Notes
	MUSCLE SPASM RELEASES – MYOFASCIAL RELEASE						
#A1	Neck Release	1	2	10 secs		nil	
#A5	Hips and ITB	1	1	15 secs		nil	
#A6	Buttocks and Piriformis	1	1	20 secs		nil	
#A7	Calf	1	1	15 secs		nil	
	STRETCHES						
#B1	Neck – Back	1	1	10 secs		nil	
#B5	Neck – Front	1	1	10 secs		nil	
#B7	Upper Back	1	1	10 secs		nil	
#B10	Lower Back	1	1	20 secs		nil	
	STABILITY						
#C3	Hip Extension – Swiss Ball	1	10	323		30 secs	
#C6	Basic 4 Point Kneeling	1	10	10 secs		nil	
	WEIGHTS GYM SESSION 3x PER WEEK						
#D1	Calf Raises	2	10	213	bodyweight	30 secs	
#D3	Swiss Ball Wall Squats	2	10	312	bodyweight	30 secs	
#D33	Push-ups – Knees	2	10	312	bodyweight	60 secs	
#D14	Rotational Lunge	1	12	202	2kg	30 secs	
#D22	Seated Row	2	12	213	light	30 secs	Use Swiss ball
#D40	DB Bicep Curls	1	20	213	2kg	30 secs	
#D42	DB Lateral Raise	1	20	213	2kg	30 secs	
#D45	Tricep Pushdown	1	20	213	light	nil	

Notes:

As you become stronger and more confident, increase repetitions of each exercise to 20.

This program can be repeated 3 times a week. On alternate days choose to walk or do a Pilates or yoga class.

PROGRAM 4

BEFORE PREGNANCY FOR BEGINNER TO INTERMEDIATE – PROGRAM 1

GYM WORKOUT
TRAINING AGE: 6-12 MONTHS
DURATION: 6 WEEKS TO 3 MONTHS

Exercise	Exercise	Sets	Reps	Tempo/Hold	Weight	Rest	Notes
MUSCLE SPASM RELEASES – MYOFASCIAL RELEASE							
#A3	Rhomboids	1	1	10 secs		nil	
#A5	Hips and ITB	1	1	15 secs		nil	
#A6	Buttocks and Piriformis	1	1	20 secs		nil	
#A8	Shins	1	1	20 secs		nil	
STRETCHES							
#B2	Neck – Side	1	1	10 secs			
#B3	Neck – Front	1	1	10 secs			
#B8	Lower Back	1	1	10 secs			
#B12	Russian Twist	1	10 total	313			
#B13	Hip and Thigh	1	1	10 secs			
STABILITY							
#C2	Hip Extension – Alternate Leg	1	10	323		30 secs	
#C9	Leg Lift – Swiss Ball	1	10	222		30 secs	
#C10	Prone Cobra – Swiss Ball	1	10	222		nil	
#C11	Lateral Ball Roll	1 to 2	8	slow		60 secs	
WEIGHTS							
#D5	Single Arm Dead Row	2-3	10	323	light	30 secs	Intermediate – do fronts squat
#D17	Torso Cable Rotation	2-3	12	213	light	60 secs	
#D24	Prone Jack Knife	2-3	12	213	bodyweight	60 secs	
#D27	Obliques – Side Crunch	2-3	10-20	213	bodyweight	60 secs	
#D38	Chest Press – Swiss Ball	2-3	20	312	2kg	60 secs	
#D39	DB Chest Flyes	2-3	12	312	2kg	60 secs	

Notes:

Regress or progress with your weights. Go at your own pace and increase sets or repetitions when you have good technique.

Cardio may be done after weights for 10-20 minutes or on another day for 30 minutes.

PROGRAM 5

BEFORE PREGNANCY FOR BEGINNER TO INTERMEDIATE – PROGRAM 2

GYM WORKOUT
TRAINING AGE: 6-12 MONTHS
DURATION: 6 WEEKS TO 3 MONTHS

Exercise	Exercise	Sets	Reps	Tempo/Hold	Weight	Rest	Notes
	MUSCLE SPASM RELEASES – MYOFASCIAL RELEASE						
#A1	Neck Release	1	2	10 secs		nil	
#A2	Latissimus Dorsi	1	2	10 secs		nil	
#A5	Hips and ITB	1	1	15 secs		nil	
#A6	Buttocks and Piriformis	1	1	20 secs		nil	
#A7	Calf	1	1	10 secs		nil	
	STRETCHES						
#B4	Neck – Side	1	1	10 secs			
#B5	Neck – Front	1	1	10 secs			
#B10	Lower Back	1	1	20 secs			
#B12	Russian Twist	1	10 total	313			
#B13	Hip and Thigh	1	1	10 secs			
	STABILITY						
#C2	Hip Extension – Alternate Leg	2	10	323		30 secs	
#C11	Lateral Ball Roll	1-2	8 total	slow		60 secs	
	WEIGHTS						
#D14	Rotational Lunge	2-3	12	202	3kg	30 secs	
#D8	Leg Press Machine	2-3	20	312	light-medium	60 secs	
#D22	Seated Row	2-3	12	213	medium	60 secs	
#D23	Seated High Row	2-3	12	213	medium	60 secs	
#D42	DB Lateral Raise	2-3	20	213	2kg	60 secs	
#D44	Tricep Dips	2-3	20	312		60 secs	
#D28	Crunches – Swiss Ball	2-3	10	213		60 secs	

Notes:

Regress or progress with your weights. Go at your own pace and increase sets or repetitions when you have good technique.

Cardio may be done after weights for 10-20 minutes or on another day for 30 minutes.

PROGRAM 6

BEFORE PREGNANCY FOR BEGINNER TO INTERMEDIATE – PROGRAM 3

GYM WORKOUT
TRAINING AGE: 6-12 MONTHS
DURATION: 6 WEEKS TO 3 MONTHS

Exercise	Exercise	Sets	Reps	Tempo/Hold	Weight	Rest	Notes
MUSCLE SPASM RELEASES – MYOFASCIAL RELEASE							
#A1	Neck Release	1	2	10 secs		nil	
#A3	Rhomboids	1	1	10 secs		nil	
#A5	Hips and ITB	2	1	15 secs		nil	
#A6	Buttocks and Piriformis	2	1	20 secs		nil	
STRETCHES							
#B3	Neck – Front	1	1	10 secs			
#B4	Neck – Side	1	1	10 secs			
#B10	Lower Back	1	1	20 secs			
#B13	Hip and Thigh	1	1	10 secs			
STABILITY							
#C2	Hip Extension – Alternate Leg	2	10	323		30 secs	
#C9	Leg Lift – Swiss Ball	1	10	222		30 secs	Try lifting both legs together
#C11	Lateral Ball Roll	1-2	8	slow		60 secs	
WEIGHTS							
#D10	Lunge on Two BOSU®	2-3	12	313	bodyweight	60 secs	beginners – no BOSU® please
#D33	Push-ups – Knees	2-3	15	312	bodyweight	60 secs	
#D18	Wood Chop	2-3	12	213	light	60 secs	
#D20	Prone Cobra	2	12	222	bodyweight	60 secs	
#D45	Tricep Pushdown	3	15-20	213	light	nil	Do this back to back with overhead tricep extension.
#D46	Tricep Extension	3	12	213	light	60 secs	
#D24	Prone Jack Knife	2-3	12-20	213	bodyweight	60 secs	Beginner – 4 point kneeling

Notes:

There is a lot of volume in this program, so only do it once a week.

Only increase sets when you have a good technique and you feel safe.

This is a great program to learn to be focused and efficient in the gym. Take your rest with stop watch, and set up for the next exercise during your rest.

PROGRAM 7

BEFORE PREGNANCY FOR BEGINNER TO INTERMEDIATE – PROGRAM 4

HOME WORKOUT
TRAINING AGE: 6-12 MONTHS
DURATION: 6 WEEKS TO 3 MONTHS

Exercise	Exercise	Sets	Reps	Tempo/Hold	Weight	Rest	Notes
	MUSCLE SPASM RELEASES – MYOFASCIAL RELEASE ON FOAM ROLLER						
#A1	Neck Release	1	2	10 secs		nil	
#A4	Lower Back	2	1	20 secs		30 secs	
#A6	Buttocks and Piriformis	1	1	20 secs		nil	
	STRETCHES						
#B2	Neck – Side	1	1	10 secs		nil	
#B5	Neck – Front	1	1	10 secs		nil	
#B7	Upper Back	1	1	10 secs		nil	
#B12	Russian Twist	1	10 total	313		nil	
	STABILITY						
#C2	Hip Extension – Alternate Leg	1	10	5 secs		30 secs	
#C7	4 Point Kneeling – Opposite Arm and Leg	1	10	424		60 secs	With extension
#C10	Prone Cobra – Swiss Ball	1	10	222		60 secs	
#C11	Lateral Ball Roll	1	8	slow		nil	
	WEIGHTS						
#D3	Swiss Ball Wall Squats	2	25	313	bodyweight	60 secs	
#D6	Hip Extension – Swiss Ball	2	20	213	bodyweight	60 secs	
#D22	Seated Row	2	12	213	medium tube	60 secs	
#D33	Push-ups – Knees	2	15	312	bodyweight	60 secs	
#D14	Rotational Lunge	2	8	202	2kg	60 secs	
#D24	Prone Jack Knife	2	12	213	bodyweight	60 secs	
#D27	Obliques – Side Crunch	2	20	213	bodyweight	60 secs	

Notes:

Increase sets to 3 when you have a good technique and you feel safe.

PROGRAM 8

BEFORE PREGNANCY FOR BEGINNER TO INTERMEDIATE – PROGRAM 5

HOME WORKOUT
TRAINING AGE: 6-12 MONTHS
DURATION: 6 WEEKS TO 3 MONTHS

Exercise	Exercise	Sets	Reps	Tempo/ Hold	Weight	Rest	Notes
MUSCLE SPASM RELEASES – MYOFASCIAL RELEASE ON FOAM ROLLER							
#A1	Neck Release	1	2	10 secs			
#A4	Lower Back	2	1	20 secs			
#A6	Buttocks and Piriformis	1	1	20 secs			
#A7	Calf	1	1	10-15 secs			
#A9	Front Thigh	1	1	15 secs			
CARDIO AND WEIGHTS: MOVE QUICKLY FROM ONE EXERCISE TO THE NEXT KEEPING HEART RATE ELEVATED.							
#DC1	Cardio Step-up	1	10 each leg	each leg		nil	
#D3	Swiss Ball Wall Squats	1	25	312	bodyweight	nil	Followed by Cardio Step-ups #DC1
#D33	Push-ups – Knees	1	12	312	bodyweight	nil	Followed by Cardio Step-ups #DC1
#D22	Seated Row	1	12	312	light tube	nil	Followed by Cardio Step-ups #DC1
#D40	DB Bicep Curls	1	10	213	2kg	nil	
#D42	DB Lateral Raise	1	10	213	2kg	nil	
#D44	Tricep Dips	1	12	312	bench	nil	Followed by Cardio Step-ups #DC1
#D9	Lunge – Swiss Ball on Wall	1	12	312	bodyweight	nil	Followed by Cardio Step-ups #DC1
#D15	Rotational Lunge and Extension	1	8	202	2kg	nil	Followed by Cardio Step-ups #DC1
#D24	Prone Jack Knife	1	12	213	bodyweight	nil	Followed by Cardio Step-ups #DC1
#D24	Prone Jack Knife	1	12	213	bodyweight	nil	
STRETCHES: CHOOSE YOUR FAVOURITE STRETCHES FOR 10 MINUTES.							

Notes:

Stepping should be medium intensity, get faster as you get fitter. However, watch your heels, and be sure you are stepping with your whole foot on the top of the step to prevent sore calves.

Work up to 2 risers under the step, for a step of about 20cm. Intermediate people can try the BOSU® for step-ups.

Intermediate people can repeat the weights and cardio 3 times over, with or without any rest before you start each superset.

PROGRAM 9

BEFORE PREGNANCY FOR INTERMEDIATE – PROGRAM 1

GYM WORKOUT

TRAINING AGE: 12-24 MONTHS

DURATION: 6-12 WEEKS

Exercise	Exercise	Sets	Reps	Tempo/ Hold	Weight	Rest	Notes
	MUSCLE SPASM RELEASES – MYOFASCIAL RELEASE						
#A1	Neck Release	1	2	10 secs		nil	
#A4	Lower Back	1	1	20 secs		nil	
#A6	Buttocks and Piriformis	2	1	20 secs		nil	
#A7	Calf	1	1	15 secs		nil	
	STRETCHES						
#B1	Neck – Back	1	1	20 secs		nil	
#B5	Neck – Front	1	1	10 secs		nil	
#B7	Upper Back	1	1	10 secs		nil	
#B10	Lower Back	1	1	20 secs		nil	
#B11	McKenzie Press-up	1	10	323		nil	
	STABILITY						
#C9	Leg Lift – Swiss Ball	2	10	222	bodyweight	60 secs	Both legs
#C5	Hip Extension – Inner Thigh	2	10	222	ball	60 secs	
	WEIGHTS						
#D4	Front Bar Squat	3-4	12	312	medium	60 secs	
#D12	Lunge and Lat Raise – BOSU®	2	12	312	3kg	60 secs	
#D24	Prone Jack Knife	3	12	213	medium	60 secs	
#D27	Obliques – Side Crunch	3	20	213	medium	60 secs	
#D40	DB Bicep Curls	3	12	213	medium	30 secs	
#D13	Lunge and Shoulder Press – BOSU®	3	12	313	medium	60 secs	
#D43	DB Tricep Extension on Swiss Ball	3	12	213	medium	60 secs	

PROGRAM 10

BEFORE PREGNANCY FOR INTERMEDIATE – PROGRAM 2

GYM WORKOUT
TRAINING AGE: 12-24 MONTHS
DURATION: 6-12 WEEKS

Exercise	Exercise	Sets	Reps	Tempo/Hold	Weight	Rest	Notes
	MUSCLE SPASM RELEASES – MYOFASCIAL RELEASE						
#A4	Lower Back	1	1	20 secs		nil	
#A5	Hips and ITB	1	1	15 secs		nil	
#A6	Buttocks and Piriformis	1	1	20 secs		nil	
#A3	Rhomboids	1	1	10 secs		nil	
	STRETCHES						
#B9	Lower Back	1	1	10 secs		nil	
#B12	Russian Twist	1	10 total	313		30 secs	
#B13	Hip and Thigh	1	1	10 secs		nil-30 secs	
#B1	Neck – Back	1	1	20 secs		nil	
#B5	Neck – Front	1	1	10 secs		nil	
	STABILITY						
#C7	4 Point Kneeling – Opposite Arm and Leg	1	10	424		nil	
#C11	Lateral Ball Roll	2	12 total	slow		nil	
	WEIGHTS						
#D6	Hip Extension – Swiss Ball	2	20	213		60 secs	
#D2	Calf Raises – Loaded	3	12	213	medium	60 secs	
#D8	Leg Press Machine	2	12	312	medium	60 secs	
#D19	Reverse Wood Chop	3	12	213	medium	60-90 secs	
#D22	Seated Row	3	12	213	medium	60 secs	
#D23	Seated High Row	3	12	213	medium	60 secs	
#D25	Obliques with Twist	4	16	313		60-90 secs	
#D28	Crunches – Swiss Ball	4	20	213		60 secs	

PROGRAM 11

BEFORE PREGNANCY FOR INTERMEDIATE – PROGRAM 3

GYM WORKOUT
TRAINING AGE: 12-24 MONTHS
DURATION: 6-12 WEEKS

Exercise	Exercise	Sets	Reps	Tempo/ Hold	Weight	Rest	Notes
	MUSCLE SPASM RELEASES – MYOFASCIAL RELEASE						
#A1	Neck Release	1	1	10 secs		nil	
#A5	Hips and ITB	1	1	15 secs		nil	
#A6	Buttocks and Piriformis	1	1	20 secs		nil	
#A7	Calf	1	1	15 secs		nil	
#A9	Front Thigh	1	1	15 secs		nil	
	STRETCHES						
#B7	Upper Back	1	1	10 secs		nil	
#B8	Lower Back	1	1	10 secs		nil	
#B11	McKenzie Press-up	1	10	323		nil	
#B14	Hip and Inner Thigh	1	1	60 secs		nil	
	STABILITY						
#C5	Hip Extension – Inner Thigh	2	10	222		60 secs	
#C10	Prone Cobra – Swiss Ball	2	10	222		60 secs	
#C7	4 Point Kneeling – Opposite Arm and Leg	1	10	424		nil	
	WEIGHTS						
#D38	Chest Press – Swiss Ball	3	12	312	medium	60 secs	Regress to #D35 if unstable
#D39	DB Chest Flyes	3	12	312	medium	60 secs	Regress to #D32
#D11	Lunge and Bicep Curl – BOSU®	3	12	312	medium	60 secs	
#D13	Lunge and Shoulder Press – BOSU®	3	12	313	medium	60 secs	
#D43	DB Tricep Extension on Swiss Ball	3	12	213	medium-light	60 secs	
#D7	Single Leg Curl – Swiss Ball	3	12	213		60 secs	Regress to using both legs
#D26	Oblique Twist – With Tuck	2-4	16	212		60-90 secs	

Notes:

You may wish to finish off with 10 mins on the bike with medium-light intensity.

You can also stretch major muscle groups e.g. legs and chest to finish.

PROGRAM 12

BEFORE PREGNANCY FOR INTERMEDIATE TO ADVANCED – PROGRAM 1

GYM WORKOUT
TRAINING AGE: 24 MONTHS ONWARDS
DURATION: 6 WEEKS

Exercise	Exercise	Sets	Reps	Tempo/ Hold	Weight	Rest	Notes
	MUSCLE SPASM RELEASES – MYOFASCIAL RELEASE						
#A1	Neck Release	1	1	10 secs		nil	
#A2	Latissimus Dorsi	1	1	10 secs		nil	
#A3	Rhomboids	1	1	10 secs		nil	
#A6	Buttocks and Piriformis	1	1	20 secs		nil	
	STRETCHES						
#B2	Neck – Side	1	1	10 secs		nil	
#B3	Neck – Front	1	1	10 secs		nil	
#B9	Lower Back	1	1	10 secs		nil	
#B10	Lower Back	1	1	20 secs		nil	
#B12	Russian Twist	1	10	313		nil	
	STABILITY						
#C2	Hip Extension – Alternate Leg	1	10	5 sec hold		nil	
#C11	Lateral Ball Roll	2	12 total	slow		60 secs	
	WEIGHTS						
#D18	Wood Chop	3	12	213	medium-heavy	60-90 secs	
#D21	Single Arm Row	3	12	213	medium-heavy	60-90 secs	
#D23	Seated High Row	3	12	213	medium-heavy	60-90 secs	
#D29	Abdominal Pike	3	12	123	bodyweight	60 secs	
#D26	Oblique Twist – With Tuck	2-4	16	212	bodyweight	60-90 secs	
#D11	Lunge and Bicep Curl – BOSU®	3	12	312	medium	60 secs	
#D13	Lunge and Shoulder Press – BOSU®	3	12	313	medium	60 secs	

PROGRAM 13
BEFORE PREGNANCY FOR INTERMEDIATE TO ADVANCED – PROGRAM 2
GYM WORKOUT
TRAINING AGE: 24 MONTHS ONWARDS
DURATION: 6 WEEKS

Exercise	Exercise	Sets	Reps	Tempo/Hold	Weight	Rest	Notes
MUSCLE SPASM RELEASES – MYOFASCIAL RELEASE							
#A4	Lower Back	1	1	20 secs		nil	
#A5	Hips and ITB	1	1	15 secs		nil	
#A6	Buttocks and Piriformis	1	1	20 secs		nil	
#A7	Calf	1	1	15 secs		nil	
#A8	Shins	1	1	10 secs		nil	
STRETCHES							
#B1	Neck – Back	1	1	20 secs		nil	
#B5	Neck – Front	1	1	10 secs		nil	
#B7	Upper Back	1	1	10 secs		nil	
#B13	Hip and Thigh	1	1	10 secs		nil	
STABILITY							
#C11	Lateral Ball Roll	1	12	slow		nil	
#C2	Hip Extension – Alternate Leg	1	10	explosive		nil	Both legs
WEIGHTS							
#D4	Front Bar Squat	4	12	312	medium-heavy	90 secs	
#D7	Single Leg Curl – Swiss Ball	2	12	213	bodyweight	60 secs	
#D35	Push-ups – Swiss Ball	3	12	312	bodyweight	60 secs	Split 6 on each leg
#D39	DB Chest Flyes	3	12	312	medium	60 secs	
#D19	Reverse Wood Chop	3	12	213	medium	60 secs	
#D46	Tricep Extension	3	12	213	medium	60 secs	
#D25	Obliques with Twist	2-4	20-30	313	bodyweight	60 secs	

PROGRAM 14

BEFORE PREGNANCY FOR INTERMEDIATE TO ADVANCED – PROGRAM 3

GYM WORKOUT
TRAINING AGE: 24 MONTHS ONWARDS
DURATION: 6 WEEKS

Exercise	Exercise	Sets	Reps	Tempo/ Hold	Weight	Rest	Notes
	MUSCLE SPASM RELEASES – MYOFASCIAL RELEASE						
#A1	Neck Release	1	1	10 secs		nil	
#A2	Latissimus Dorsi	1	1	10 secs		nil	
#A3	Rhomboids	1	1	10 secs		nil	
#A5	Hips and ITB	1	1	15 secs		nil	
#A6	Buttocks and Piriformis	1	1	20 secs		nil	
	STRETCHES						
#B7	Upper Back	1	1	10 secs		nil	
#B9	Lower Back	1	1	10 secs		nil	
#B12	Russian Twist	1	10 total	10 secs		nil	
#B13	Hip and Thigh	2	1	10 secs		nil	
	STABILITY						
#C11	Lateral Ball Roll	1	12	slow		nil	
#C10	Prone Cobra – Swiss Ball	1	10	222		nil	
	WEIGHTS						
#D5	Single Arm Dead Row	3	12	312	medium-heavy	60-90 secs	Pull for 12 reps on each arm
#D23	Seated High Row	3	12	213	medium	60 secs	
#D8	Leg Press Machine	2 to 4	12	312	medium-heavy	60-90 secs	
#D36	DB Chest Press – Bench	3	12	312	medium-heavy	60 secs	
#D40	DB Bicep Curls	2	12	213	medium-heavy	60 secs	
#D42	DB Lateral Raise	2	12	213	medium-heavy	60 secs	
#D46	Tricep Extension	2	12	213	medium-heavy	60 secs	
#D29	Abdominal Pike	3	12	123	bodyweight	60 secs	
#D26	Oblique Twist – With Tuck	2	16	212	bodyweight	60 secs	

Notes:

Do not stretch after weights. When muscles are shortened by strengthening, you don't want to stretch them by lengthening them.

PROGRAM 15

1ST TRIMESTER EXERCISE PROGRAM – PROGRAM 1

GYM WORKOUT – BEGINNER AND REGULAR EXERCISER

COMBINED CARDIO AND WEIGHTS

Exercise	Exercise	Sets	Reps	Tempo/ Hold	Weight	Rest	Notes
MUSCLE SPASM RELEASES – MYOFASCIAL RELEASE							
#E1	Foot – Golf Ball	1		10 secs	5/10	nil	
#E3	ITB – Foam Roller	2		15 secs	6/10	nil	
STRETCHES							
#F1	Calf – Wall	1		20 secs		nil	
#F3	Hamstrings	1		20 secs		nil	
#F4	Inner Thigh	1		20 secs		nil	
#F5	Piriformis – Hip	1		20 secs		nil	Right leg, Left leg x 2
#F8	Hip Flexor – Kneeling	1		20 secs		nil	
#F11	Chest	1		20 secs		nil	
#F12	Latissimus	1		20 secs		nil	
#F14	Neck – Back	1		20 secs		nil	
MOBILITY AND STABILITY							
#G4	Russian Twist	1	10 total	313		30 secs	
#H2	4 Point Kneeling	1	10	10 secs		60 secs	
WEIGHTS							
#H7	Swiss Ball Wall Squat	2	15	313		nil	Cardio Step ups #DC1 after each set
#H14	Standing Tube Row	2	15	313		nil	Cardio Step ups #DC1 after each set
#H1	Bridge on the Swiss Ball	2	10	312		nil	Cardio Step ups #DC1 after each set
#H10	Rotational Lunge	2	8	202		nil	Cardio Step ups #DC1 after each set
#H12	Chest Press – Swiss Ball	2	15	312		nil	Cardio Step ups #DC1 after each set
#H16	DB Bicep Curl	2	10	313		nil	Cardio Step ups #DC1 after each set

Notes:

If you exercise regularly, increase to 3 sets in your weights section.

Monitor your heart rate and exertion level.

PROGRAM 16

1ST TRIMESTER EXERCISE PROGRAM – PROGRAM 2

GYM WORKOUT – BEGINNER AND REGULAR EXERCISER

WEIGHTS DAY ONLY – NO CARDIO

Exercise	Exercise	Sets	Reps	Tempo/ Hold	Weight	Rest	Notes
MUSCLE SPASM RELEASES – MYOFASCIAL RELEASE							
#E3	ITB – Foam Roller	1		20 secs	6/10	nil	
WARM-UP							
	Bike, Treadmill or Cross Trainer	1	5 minutes	warm up			
STRETCHES							
#F1	Calf – Wall	1	1	20 secs		nil	
#F3	Hamstrings	1	1	20 secs		nil	
#F5	Piriformis – Hip	2	1	20 secs		nil	
#F6	Quadriceps	1	1	20 secs		nil	
STABILITY							
#G4	Russian Twist	2	10 total	313	bodyweight	60 secs	
#G6	Hip Extensions – Swiss Ball	2	12	222		60 secs	
WEIGHTS							
#H7	Swiss Ball Wall Squat	3	20	313	bodyweight	60 secs	
#H12	Chest Press – Swiss Ball	3	20	312	2-5kg	60 secs	Start with light weight
#H15	Seated Row	3	15	213	light-medium	60 secs	Cable machine
#H6	Leg Curls with Swiss Ball	3	10	313	ball only	60 secs	
#H5	4 Point Kneeling – Arm and Leg	2	10	controlled		60 secs	10 second contraction

Notes:

For beginners use 2kg dumbbells, regular exercisers should use 5kg for chest and 3-4kg for bicep curls.

PROGRAM 17

1ST TRIMESTER EXERCISE PROGRAM – PROGRAM 3

GYM WORKOUT – BEGINNER AND REGULAR EXERCISER

STRETCH AND CARDIO

Exercise	Exercise	Sets	Reps	Tempo/ Hold	Weight	Rest	Notes
MUSCLE SPASM RELEASES – MYOFASCIAL RELEASE							
#E3	ITB – Foam Roller	2	1	20 secs	6/10	nil	
PRE-STRETCH							
#F1	Calf – Wall	1	1	20 secs		nil	
#F2	Achilles – Wall/Chair Version	1	1	20 secs		nil	
#F3	Hamstrings	1	1	20 secs		nil	
#F4	Inner Thigh	1	1	20 secs		nil	
#F5	Piriformis – Hip	2	1	20 secs		nil	
#F8	Hip Flexor – Kneeling	1	1	20 secs		nil	
#F10	Lower Back and Waist	1	1	20 secs		nil	
#F11	Chest	1	1	20 secs		nil	
CARDIO							
	Bike	1	10 mins				Intensity should be RPE 13-14
	Treadmill	1	10 mins				Intensity should be RPE 13-14
	Cross Trainer	1	10 mins				Intensity should be RPE 13-14
FOLLOWED BY							
#H19	Blood Pressure Cuff	2	10	10 secs		60 secs	
#H5	4 Point Kneeling – Arm and Leg	2	10	10 secs		60 secs	
POST-CARDIO STRETCH							
#F6	Quadriceps	1	1	30 secs		nil	
#F3	Hamstrings	1	1	30 secs		nil	
#F4	Inner Thigh	1	1	30 secs		nil	
#F5	Piriformis – Hip	1	1	30 secs		nil	
#F14	Neck – Back	1	1	30 secs		nil	30 secs each side

Notes:

Keep your heart rate within your range and intensity at the recommended level.

PROGRAM 18

1ST TRIMESTER EXERCISE PROGRAM – PROGRAM 4

GYM WORKOUT – BEGINNER AND REGULAR EXERCISER

WEIGHTS DAY

Exercise	Exercise	Sets	Reps	Tempo/ Hold	Weight	Rest	Notes
	MUSCLE SPASM RELEASES – MYOFASCIAL RELEASE						
#E3	ITB – Foam Roller	2		20 seconds		nil	
	STABILITY						
#G1	Lateral Pelvic Tilt	1	20 total	slow		nil	
#G2	Anterior & Posterior Pelvic Tilt	1	20 total	slow		nil	
#G9	Buttock Squeeze -Tube	1	10 each side	212		nil	
#G8	Hip Extension – Towel	1	10	323		nil	Or 2kg medicine ball
#G4	Russian Twist	1	10	313		nil	
	WEIGHTS						
#H6	Leg Curls with Swiss Ball	1	10	313		nil	No rest-move on to the next
#H8	Ball Squats – Med Ball	1	20	313		nil	exercise and keep going
#H12	Chest Press – Swiss Ball	1	20	312	2-5kg DB	nil	until finished with standing
#H10	Rotational Lunge	1	12	202	0-2kg MB	nil	row.
#H13	Single Arm Row	1	15	213	medium	nil	Followed with a quick 5 min
#H19	Blood Pressure Cuff	1	10	414		nil	stretch of major
#H16	DB Bicep Curl	1	10 each leg	313	2kg DB	nil	muscle groups.
#H17	Lateral Raises on Swiss Ball	1	10 each leg	213	2kg DB	nil	
#H18	Shoulder Press	1	15	312	2kg DB	nil	
#H14	Standing Tube Row	1	15	213	medium	nil	

Notes:

If your feet are on the floor for Biceps, Lateral Raise and Shoulder Press, do a total of 20 repetitions. Choose your weight appropriately.

This program has weights with no rest period and covers whole body training.

PROGRAM 19

1ST TRIMESTER EXERCISE PROGRAM – PROGRAM 5
HOME WORKOUT – BEGINNER
STRETCHES WITH 20 MINUTE WALK

Exercise	Exercise	Sets	Reps	Intensity	Hold	Rest	Notes
	MUSCLE SPASM RELEASES – MYOFASCIAL RELEASE						
#E1	Foot – Golf Ball	1	1	5/10	10 secs	nil	
#E2	Shins – Towel Grip	1	10	5/10	N/A	nil	
#E3	ITB – Foam Roller	1	1	6/10	15 secs	nil	
#E4	Lats and Shoulders – Foam Roller	1	1	6/10	10 secs	nil	
	STRETCHES						
#F1	Calf – Wall	1	1		20 secs	nil	
#F2	Achilles – Wall/Chair Version	1	1		20 secs	nil	
#F3	Hamstrings	1	1		20 secs	nil	
#F4	Inner Thigh	1	1		20 secs	nil	
#F5	Piriformis – Hip	2	1		20 secs	nil	
#F6	Quadriceps	1	1		20 secs	nil	
#F8	Hip Flexor – Kneeling	1	1		10-20 secs	nil	
#F9	Side Leg	1	1		10 secs	nil	
#F10	Lower Back and Waist	1	1		10-20 secs	nil	
#F11	Chest	1	1		20 secs	nil	
#F12	Latissimus	1	1		20 secs	nil	
#F14	Neck – Back	1	1		20 secs	nil	
#F15	Neck – Side and Front	1	1		20 secs	nil	
#F16	Neck – Back	1	1		20 secs	nil	

Notes:

Follow this with a 20 minute walk and a quick 5 minute calf, hamstring and quadriceps stretch.

Monitor your heart rate, and write it down, so you can keep track of it.

Remember that week 8-13 your baby's organs are forming – so do not exert your heart rate above 140 beats per minute.

PROGRAM 20

1ST TRIMESTER EXERCISE PROGRAM – PROGRAM 6

HOME WORKOUT – BEGINNER STRETCHES WITH 20 MINUTE WALK

Exercise	Exercise	Sets	Reps	Intensity	Tempo/ Hold	Rest	Notes
MUSCLE SPASM RELEASES – MYOFASCIAL RELEASE							
#E1	Foot – Golf Ball	1	1	5/10	10 secs	nil	
#E3	ITB – Foam Roller	2	1	6/10	15 secs	nil	do each thigh twice
STRETCHES							
#F1	Calf – Wall	1	1		20 secs	nil	
#F3	Hamstrings	1	1		20 secs	nil	
#F5	Piriformis – Hip	2	1		20 secs	nil	
#F7	Hip Flexor – Standing	1	1		20 secs	nil	
#F11	Chest	1	1		20 secs	nil	
#F13	Back	1	1		10 secs	nil	
#F14	Neck – Back	1	1		20 secs	nil	
STABILITY							
#G8	Hip Extension – Towel	1	10		323	nil	
#G9	Buttock Squeeze -Tube	1	10		213	nil	
WEIGHTS							
#H7	Swiss Ball Wall Squat	2	20	313	bodyweight	60 secs	
#H12	Chest Press – Swiss Ball	2	20	312	2-4kgDB	60 secs	
#H14	Standing Tube Row	2	15	213	light-medium	60 secs	
#H16	DB Bicep Curl	2	10 each leg	313	0-2kg DB	60 secs	Start with no weight
#H17	Lateral Raises on Swiss Ball	2	20 total	213	0-2kg DB	60 secs	10 on each leg
#H18	Shoulder Press	2	15	213	0-2kg DB	60 secs	
#H5	4 Point Kneeling – Arm and Leg	2	10 total	213	nil	60 secs	

PROGRAM 21
1ST TRIMESTER EXERCISE PROGRAM – PROGRAM 7
HOME WORKOUT – BEGINNER
MIX OF WEIGHTS AND CARDIO

Exercise	Exercise	Sets	Reps	Tempo/ Hold	Weight	Rest	Notes
MUSCLE SPASM RELEASES – MYOFASCIAL RELEASE							
#E3	ITB – Foam Roller	2	1	15 secs	6/10	nil	Do each thigh twice
#E4	Lats and Shoulders – Foam Roller	1	1	10 secs	6/10	nil	
STRETCHES							
#F1	Calf – Wall	1	1	20 secs		nil	
#F11	Chest	1	1	20 secs		nil	
#F8	Hip Flexor – Kneeling	1	1	20 secs		nil	
#F4	Inner Thigh	1	1	20 secs		nil	
#F3	Hamstrings	1	1	20 secs		nil	
WEIGHTS AND CARDIO							
#H1	Bridge on the Swiss Ball	2	10	312	nil	nil	Cardio Step ups #DC1 after each set
#H10	Rotational Lunge	2	8	202	nil	nil	Cardio Step ups #DC1 after each set
#H12	Chest Press – Swiss Ball	2	20	312	2kg	nil	Cardio Step ups #DC1 after each set
#H7	Swiss Ball Wall Squat	2	20	313	nil	nil	Cardio Step ups #DC1 after each set
#H15	Seated Row	2	20	312	tube	nil	Cardio Step ups #DC1 after each set
#H17	Lateral Raises on Swiss Ball	2	20	213	2kg	nil	Cardio Step ups #DC1 after each set

Notes:

You can use a commercial step or any kind of solid step that you have in your home. If you don't have a step, use the first step of your stairs in your home – but make sure it is safe.

PROGRAM 22

1ST TRIMESTER EXERCISE PROGRAM – PROGRAM 8
HOME WORKOUT – BEGINNER
CORE – STABILITY, MOBILITY AND STRENGTH

Exercise	Exercise	Sets	Reps	Tempo/ Hold	Weight	Rest	Notes
MUSCLE SPASM RELEASES – MYOFASCIAL RELEASE							
#E1	Foot – Golf Ball	1	1	10 secs	5/10	nil	Do each thigh twice
#E3	ITB – Foam Roller	2	1	15 secs	6/10	nil	
STRETCHES							
#F1	Calf – Wall	1	1	20 secs	nil	nil	
#F11	Chest	1	1	20 secs	nil	nil	
#F8	Hip Flexor – Kneeling	1	1	20 secs	nil	nil	
#F4	Inner Thigh	1	1	20 secs	nil	nil	
#F3	Hamstrings	1	1	20 secs	nil	nil	
STABILITY AND MOBILITY							
#G1	Lateral Pelvic Tilt	1	20 total	controlled	nil	nil	Move in a controlled manner
#G2	Anterior & Posterior Pelvic Tilt	1	20 total	controlled	nil	nil	
#G4	Russian Twist	3	10 each side	313	nil	60 secs	Move in a controlled manner
#G6	Hip Extensions – Swiss Ball	2	12	222	nil	60 secs	
#G9	Buttock Squeeze -Tube	3	10	213	nil	60 secs	Controlled contraction
WEIGHTS							
#H6	Leg Curls with Swiss Ball	2	10	312	nil	60 secs	
#H13	Single Arm Row	2	15	213	light tube	60 secs	
#H5	4 Point Kneeling – Arm and Leg	2	10	slow	nil	60 secs	

Notes:

Exercise #H5: regress to 1 arm and 1 leg if you are losing form.

PROGRAM 23
2ND TRIMESTER EXERCISE PROGRAM – PROGRAM 1
HOME OR GYM WORKOUT
WEIGHTS AND CARDIO WORKOUT

Exercise	Exercise	Sets	Reps	Tempo/Hold	Weight	Rest	Notes
	MUSCLE SPASM RELEASES – MYOFASCIAL RELEASE						
#E1	Foot – Golf Ball	1		10 secs	5/10	nil	
#E3	ITB – Foam Roller	2		15 secs	6/10	nil	
	STRETCHES						
#F1	Calf – Wall	1		20 secs		nil	
#F3	Hamstrings	1		20 secs		nil	
#F4	Inner Thigh	1		20 secs		nil	
#F5	Piriformis – Hip	1		20 secs		nil	
#F8	Hip Flexor – Kneeling	1		20 secs		nil	
#F10	Lower Back and Waist	1		20 secs		nil	
#F14	Neck – Back	1		20 secs		nil	
	MOBILITY AND STABILITY						
#G1	Lateral Pelvic Tilt	1	20 total	slow		nil	
#G2	Anterior & Posterior Pelvic Tilt	1	20 total	slow		nil	
#G4	Russian Twist	1	10 total	slow		nil	
#G7	Hip Extension – Floor	1	10 total	slow		nil	
	WEIGHTS						
#H6	Leg Curls with Swiss Ball	2	10	313		60 secs	
#H8	Ball Squats – Med Ball	3	12	313		nil	Cardio Step ups #DC1 after each set
#H13	Single Arm Row	3	15	213		nil	Cardio Step ups #DC1 after each set
#H17	Lateral Raises on Swiss Ball	3	15	213	2kg	nil	Cardio Step ups #DC1 after each set
#H18	Shoulder Press	3	15	213	2kg	nil	Cardio Step ups #DC1 after each set
#H19	Blood Pressure Cuff	3	10	10 secs	40-60 mmHg	60 secs	Roll on to your left for rest

Notes:

Only use the platform for stepping up and down. Keep your heart rate within your range.

Weights and cardio combined in the session with no rest period is a great way to combine resistance and cardio workout.

PROGRAM 24
2ND TRIMESTER EXERCISE PROGRAM – PROGRAM 2
HOME OR GYM WORKOUT
WEIGHTS AND CARDIO WORKOUT

Exercise	Exercise	Sets	Reps	Tempo/Hold	Weight	Rest	Notes
	MUSCLE SPASM RELEASES – MYOFASCIAL RELEASE						
#E1	Foot – Golf Ball	1		10 secs	5/10	nil	
#E3	ITB – Foam Roller	2		15 secs	6/10	nil	
	STRETCHES						
#F1	Calf – Wall	1		20 secs		nil	
#F3	Hamstrings	1		20 secs		nil	
#F4	Inner Thigh	1		20 secs		nil	
#F5	Piriformis – Hip	1		20 secs		nil	
#F8	Hip Flexor – Kneeling	1		20 secs		nil	
#F10	Lower Back and Waist	1		20 secs		nil	
#F14	Neck – Back	1		20 secs		nil	
	MOBILITY AND STABILITY						
#G1	Lateral Pelvic Tilt	1	20 total	slow		nil	
#G2	Anterior & Posterior Pelvic Tilt	1	20 total	slow		nil	
#G4	Russian Twist	1	10 total	slow		nil	
#G7	Hip Extension – Floor	1	10 total	slow		nil	
	CARDIO ONLY						
	Walk		30 mins				Medium intensity
	OR split into						
	Treadmill		10 mins				Medium intensity
	Bike		10 mins				Medium intensity
	Cross-Trainer		10 mins				Medium intensity

Notes:

Stretch major muscle groups for 5 minutes after cardio.

PROGRAM 25
2ND TRIMESTER EXERCISE PROGRAM – PROGRAM 3
HOME OR GYM WORKOUT

Exercise	Exercise	Sets	Reps	Tempo/ Hold	Weight	Rest	Notes
				MUSCLE SPASM RELEASES – MYOFASCIAL RELEASE			
	As needed						
				STRETCHES			
#F4	Inner Thigh	1		20 secs		nil	
#F8	Hip Flexor – Kneeling	1		20 secs		nil	
#F5	Piriformis – Hip	2		10 secs		nil	
				STABILITY			
#G1	Lateral Pelvic Tilt	1	20 total	slow		nil	
#G2	Anterior & Posterior Pelvic Tilt	1	20 total	slow		nil	
#G4	Russian Twist	1	10 total	slow		nil	
#G7	Hip Extension – Floor	1	10 total	slow		nil	
				WEIGHTS			
#H10	Rotational Lunge	2	12	202	2kg	60 secs	Only if comfortable
#H9	Side-on Swiss Ball Squats	3	10	313		60 secs	
#H12	Chest Press – Swiss Ball	3	20	312	2-5kg	60 secs	
#H13	Single Arm Row	3	15	213	medium	60 secs	
#H19	Blood Pressure Cuff	2	10	10 sec hold	40-50 mmHg	60 secs	Roll on to left side during rest
#H3	4 Point Kneeling – Leg	2	10	313	bodyweight	60 secs	

PROGRAM 26
2ND TRIMESTER EXERCISE PROGRAM – PROGRAM 4
HOME OR GYM WORKOUT
WEIGHTS AND CARDIO WORKOUT

Exercise	Exercise	Sets	Reps	Tempo/Hold	Weight	Rest	Notes
	MUSCLE SPASM RELEASES – MYOFASCIAL RELEASE						
	As needed						
	STRETCHES						
#F3	Hamstrings	1		20 secs		nil	
#F4	Inner Thigh	1		20 secs		nil	
#F5	Piriformis – Hip	2		20 secs		nil	
#F10	Lower Back and Waist	1		20 secs		nil	
#F11	Chest	1		20 secs		nil	
	STABILITY						
#G1	Lateral Pelvic Tilt	1	20 total	slow		nil	
#G2	Anterior & Posterior Pelvic Tilt	1	20 total	slow		nil	
#G4	Russian Twist	1	10 total	slow		nil	
#G7	Hip Extension – Floor	1	10 total	slow		nil	
	WEIGHTS						
#H1	Bridge on the Swiss Ball	1	10	313		nil	
#H6	Leg Curls with Swiss Ball	2	10 to 15	213		60 secs	Perform within your comfort
#H13	Single Arm Row	2	15	213	light	60 secs	
#H12	Chest Press – Swiss Ball	2	20	312	2-5kg	60 secs	
#H10	Rotational Lunge	2	12 each side	202	2kg	60 secs	
#H7	Swiss Ball Wall Squat	2	15	313		60 secs	
	ABS						
#H19	Blood Pressure Cuff	2	10	10 secs	40-50 mmHg	60 secs	
#H5	4 Point Kneeling – Arm and Leg	2	10	slow		60 secs	

PROGRAM 27

3RD TRIMESTER EXERCISE PROGRAM – PROGRAM 1
HOME OR GYM WORKOUT
STRETCHES WITH 20 MINUTE WALK

Exercise	Exercise	Sets	Reps	Tempo/ Hold	Weight	Rest	Notes
	MUSCLE SPASM RELEASES – MYOFASCIAL RELEASE						
	nil						
	STRETCHES						
#F1	Calf – Wall	1		20 secs		nil	
#F3	Hamstrings	1		20 secs		nil	Choose a comfortable version
#F4	Inner Thigh	1		20 secs		nil	
#F5	Piriformis – Hip	1		20 secs		nil	
#F6	Quadriceps	1		20 secs		nil	Only if comfortable
#F11	Chest	1		20 secs		nil	
#F14	Neck – Back	1		20 secs		nil	
#F15	Neck – Side and Front	1		20 secs		nil	
#F16	Neck – Back	1		20 secs		nil	
#F17	Back and Breathing	1		20 secs		nil	
	STABILITY						
#G1	Lateral Pelvic Tilt	1	10 total	slow		nil	
#G2	Anterior & Posterior Pelvic Tilt	1	10 total	slow		nil	
#G5	Muscle Energy Release	1	10	controlled		nil	
	WEIGHTS						
#H5	4 Point Kneeling – Arm and Leg	2	10 total	very slow		60 secs	
	FOLLOWED BY						
	Walk		20 mins				
	FOLLOWED BY						
	Stretch major muscle groups		5 mins				

PROGRAM 28

3RD TRIMESTER EXERCISE PROGRAM – PROGRAM 2
HOME OR GYM WORKOUT
QUICK LIGHT WORKOUT

Exercise	Exercise	Sets	Reps	Tempo/Hold	Weight	Rest	Notes
	MUSCLE SPASM RELEASES – MYOFASCIAL RELEASE						
	Nil						
	STRETCHES						
#F5	Piriformis – Hip	1	1	20 sec		nil	
	STABILITY						
#G1	Lateral Pelvic Tilt	1	20	slow		nil	
#G2	Anterior & Posterior Pelvic Tilt	1	20	slow		nil	
	WEIGHTS						
#H5	4 Point Kneeling – Arm and Leg	1	10 total	313		nil	
#H7	Swiss Ball Wall Squat	1	15	313		nil	
#H12	Chest Press – Swiss Ball	1	15	312	2kg	nil	
#H13	Single Arm Row	1	15	213	light	nil	

PROGRAM 29

3RD TRIMESTER EXERCISE PROGRAM – PROGRAM 3
HOME OR GYM WORKOUT
WALK OR LIGHT WEIGHTS

Exercise	Exercise	Sets	Reps	Tempo/Hold	Weight	Rest	Notes
	MUSCLE SPASM RELEASES – MYOFASCIAL RELEASE						
	Nil						
	STRETCHES						
#F1	Calf – Wall	1		20 secs		nil	
#F3	Hamstrings	1		20 secs		nil	
#F5	Piriformis – Hip	1		20 secs		nil	
#F8	Hip Flexor – Kneeling	1		20 secs		nil	
#F11	Chest	1		20 secs		nil	
#F12	Latissimus	1		20 secs		nil	
#F17	Back and Breathing	1		20 secs		nil	
	MOBILITY AND STABILITY						
#G1	Lateral Pelvic Tilt	1	10 total	slow		nil	
#G2	Anterior & Posterior Pelvic Tilt	1	10 total	slow		nil	
#G8	Hip Extension – Towel	1	10 total	slow		nil	
	CARDIO OR WEIGHTS						
	Walk or Bike		20 mins				
	WEIGHTS OR CARDIO						
#H16	DB Bicep Curl	1	10 each leg	313	2kg	60 secs	
#H17	Lateral Raises on Swiss Ball	1	10 each leg	213	2kg	60 secs	
#H13	Single Arm Row	1	15	213	light	60 secs	
#H3	4 Point Kneeling – Leg	1	10 each leg	313	bodyweight	60 secs	

PROGRAM 30

AFTER PREGNANCY FIRST 3 MONTHS – PROGRAM 1
HOME OR GYM WORKOUT
STRETCHES, MOBILITY AND 20 MINUTE WALK

Exercise	Exercise	Sets	Reps	Tempo/Hold	Weight	Rest	Notes
				MUSCLE SPASM RELEASES – MYOFASCIAL RELEASE			
#A1	Neck Release	1		10 secs		nil	Foam Roller
#A4	Lower Back	1		10-20 secs		nil	Foam Roller
#A5	Hips and ITB	1		15 secs		nil	Foam Roller
#A6	Buttocks and Piriformis	1		20 secs		nil	Foam Roller
#A9	Front Thigh	1		20 secs		nil	Foam Roller
				STRETCHES			
#B2	Neck – Side	1		10 secs		nil	
#B6	Upper Back	1		20 secs		nil	
#B12	Russian Twist	1	10 total	slow		nil	
#B14	Hip and Inner Thigh	1		60 secs		nil	Pic 1 only
				STABILITY			
#C1	Hip Extension – Floor	2	10	323		30-60 secs	
#C6	Basic 4 Point Kneeling	2	10	10 secs		60 secs	
#C7	4 Point Kneeling – Opposite Arm and Leg	2	10 total	slow		60 secs	
				WEIGHTS			
	nil						
				CARDIO			
	Walk		20 mins				

Note: this program is from 6 weeks post delivery – after you have clearance from your OBG.

PROGRAM 31

AFTER PREGNANCY FIRST 3 MONTHS – PROGRAM 2
HOME OR GYM WORKOUT
STABILITY AND 30 MINUTE WALK

Exercise	Exercise	Sets	Reps	Tempo/Hold	Weight	Rest	Notes
	MUSCLE SPASM RELEASES – MYOFASCIAL RELEASE						
#A5	Hips and ITB	1		15 secs		nil	Foam Roller
#A6	Buttocks and Piriformis	1		20 secs		nil	Foam Roller
#A9	Front Thigh	1		20 secs		nil	Foam Roller
	STRETCHES						
	Do a quick 5 minutes stretch of the major muscles e.g. calf, thighs, hamstrings						
	STABILITY						
#C3	Hip Extension – Swiss Ball	1	10	323		nil	
#C4	Hip Extension – Outer Thigh	1	10 each side	222		nil	
#C5	Hip Extension – Inner Thigh	1	10	222		nil	
#H19	Blood Pressure Cuff	2	10	10 secs		nil	
	CARDIO						
	Walk		30 mins				
	OR AT THE GYM						
	Bike		10 mins				Intensity RPE 12-14
	Treadmill		10 mins				Intensity RPE 12-14
	Cross-Trainer or Rower		10 mins				Intensity RPE 12-14
	STRETCHES						
	Do a quick 5 minutes stretch of the major muscles e.g. calf, thighs, hamstrings						

Note: this program is from 6 weeks post delivery – after you have clearance from your OBG.

PROGRAM 32

AFTER PREGNANCY FIRST 3 MONTHS – PROGRAM 3
HOME OR GYM WORKOUT
STABILITY AND BASIC WEIGHTS

NOTE: THIS PROGRAM IS FROM 6 WEEKS POST DELIVERY – AFTER YOU HAVE CLEARANCE FROM YOUR OBG.

Exercise	Exercise	Sets	Reps	Tempo/Hold	Weight	Rest	Notes
MUSCLE SPASM RELEASES – MYOFASCIAL RELEASE							
#A1	Neck Release	1	2	10 secs		nil	
#A6	Buttocks and Piriformis	2	1	20 secs		nil	
STRETCHES							
#B2	Neck – Side	1		10 secs		nil	
#B6	Upper Back	1		20 secs		nil	
#B12	Russian Twist	1	10 total	slow		nil	
STABILITY							
#C3	Hip Extension – Swiss Ball	1	10	323		30-60secs	
#C9	Leg Lift – Swiss Ball	1	10 each leg	222		30-60 secs	
WEIGHTS							
#D1	Calf Raises	1	10	213		nil	
#D3	Swiss Ball Wall Squats	2	15-20	313		60 secs	
#D22	Seated Row	1	12	213		60 secs	At home use a tube
#D30	Push-ups – Floor	1	10	312		30 secs	Progress to #D31 on the wall
#D40	DB Bicep Curls	2	20	213	light	30 secs	
#D42	DB Lateral Raise	2	12-20	213	light	30 secs	
#D44	Tricep Dips	2	12	312		60 secs	
#C7	4 Point Kneeling – Opposite Arm and Leg	2	10	424		60 secs	

PROGRAM 33

AFTER PREGNANCY FROM 3-6 MONTHS AND ONWARDS – PROGRAM 1
HOME OR GYM WORKOUT
WEIGHTS ONLY

Exercise	Exercise	Sets	Reps	Tempo/ Hold	Weight	Rest	Notes
				MUSCLE SPASM RELEASES – MYOFASCIAL RELEASE			
	Nil						
				STABILITY – DO THIS SECTION FIRST – AS THIS IS YOUR WARM UP			
#C3	Hip Extension – Swiss Ball	2	10	323		30 secs	
#C10	Prone Cobra – Swiss Ball	2	10	222		30 secs	
#C11	Lateral Ball Roll	2	10 total	slow		30 secs	
#C7	4 Point Kneeling – Opposite Arm and Leg	1	10	424		nil	
				STRETCHES			
#B7	Upper Back	1		10 secs		nil	
#B9	Lower Back	1		10 secs		nil	
#B12	Russian Twist	1	10	313	bodyweight	nil	
#B13	Hip and Thigh	1		10 secs		nil	With or without Swiss ball
#B14	Hip and Inner Thigh	1		60 secs			
				WEIGHTS			
#D3	Swiss Ball Wall Squats	2	25	313		60 secs	
#D33	Push-ups – Knees	2	15	312		60 secs	
#D23	Seated High Row	2	12	213	light-medium	60 secs	If at home use medium tube.
#D15	Rotational Lunge and Extension	2	20 each leg	202		60 secs	
#D17	Torso Cable Rotation	2	12	213	light	60 secs	
#D24	Prone Jack Knife	2	12	213		60 secs	Only if you are ready
#D27	Obliques – Side Crunch	2	10-20	213		60 secs	Only if you are ready

Notes:

If you don't feel your core and abdominals are ready for the Prone Jack Knife and Oblique work – please regress to the 4 point kneeling, blood pressure cuff, or hovers on knees – until you feel that your back and core are strong enough.

PROGRAM 34

AFTER PREGNANCY FROM 3-6 MONTHS AND ONWARDS – PROGRAM 2
HOME OR GYM WORKOUT
CARDIO AND WEIGHTS COMBO

Exercise	Exercise	Sets	Reps	Tempo/Hold	Weight	Rest	Notes
			MUSCLE SPASM RELEASES – MYOFASCIAL RELEASE				
	As needed						
		CARDIO AND WEIGHTS COMBO – DO THIS FIRST					
#DC1	Cardio Step up	1	10 each leg	normal	bodyweight	nil	Step or BOSU®
#D5	Single Arm Dead Row	1	12 each arm	312	medium	nil	At home use a tube
	repeat this 3 x						
#DC1	Cardio Step up	1	10 each leg	normal	bodyweight	nil	Step or BOSU®
#D6	Hip Extension – Swiss Ball	1	20	213		nil	
	repeat this 3 x						
#DC1	Cardio Step up	1	10 each leg	normal	bodyweight	nil	
#D38	Chest Press – Swiss Ball	1	20	312	2-5kg	nil	Use appropriate weight
	repeat this 3 x						
#DC1	Cardio Step up	1	10 each leg	normal	body only	nil	
#D18	Wood Chop	1	12	213	medium	nil	Arms only
	repeat this 3 x						
		STRETCHES – Time permitting you can repeat each stretch					
#B15	Calf	1		30 secs		nil	
#B16	Shin	1		20 secs		nil	
#B17	Hamstring	1		30 secs		nil	
#B14	Hip and Inner Thigh	1		10 secs		nil	With or without Swiss ball
#B10	Lower Back	1		30 secs		nil	
#B6	Upper Back	1		30 secs		nil	

Notes:

Last exercise is the Wood Chop – do this as an option. If you are at home and you are not able to do it – skip it.

Focus on your deep abdominal wall and pelvic floor muscles getting stronger as this will serve you in the long run.

PROGRAM 35

AFTER PREGNANCY FROM 3-6 MONTHS AND ONWARDS – PROGRAM 3
HOME OR GYM WORKOUT
CARDIO AND WEIGHTS COMBO

Exercise	Exercise	Sets	Reps	Tempo/Hold	Weight	Rest	Notes
			MUSCLE SPASM RELEASES – MYOFASCIAL RELEASE				
	Nil						
		CARDIO AND WEIGHTS COMBO – DO THESE FIRST					
	Bike		5 mins				Warm up
#D16	Squat with DB Extension	2	12	212	2kg	nil	
	Bike		2 mins				Intensity RPE 13-14
#D21	Single Arm Row	2	12	213	light to medium	nil	
	Bike		2 mins				Intensity RPE 13-14
#D24	Prone Jack Knife	2	10	213	bodyweight	nil	
	Bike		2 mins				Intensity RPE 13-14
#D33	Push-ups – Knees	2	15	312	bodyweight	nil	
	Bike		2 mins				Intensity RPE 13-14
#D40	DB Bicep Curls	1	20	213	2-4kg	nil	do all these 3 exercises back to back with nil rest and then do the 2 min bike
#D42	DB Lateral Raise	1	20	213	2-3kg	nil	
#D44	Tricep Dips	1	20	312		nil	
	Bike		2 mins				Intensity RPE 13-14
#D6	Hip Extension – Swiss Ball	2	12 to 20	213		nil	
	Bike		2 mins				Intensity RPE 13-14
#D27	Obliques – Side Crunch	2	10 to 20	213	bodyweight	nil	
	Bike		5 mins				Cool down Intensity RPE 10-11
		STRETCHES AFTER WEIGHTS AND BIKE					
#B15	Calf	1		30 secs		nil	
#B16	Shin	1		20 secs		nil	
#B17	Hamstring	1		30 secs		nil	
#B14	Hip and Inner Thigh	1		10 secs		nil	With or without Swiss ball
#B10	Lower Back	1		30 secs		nil	
#B6	Upper Back	1		30 secs		nil	

Notes:

Intensity on the bike should be around RPE 13-14. You should be puffed out and sweating after 2 minutes.

This program increases cardiovascular fitness while toning.

PROGRAM 36

BEFORE PREGNANCY EXERCISE FOR HIP AND KNEE ISSUES
HOME OR GYM WORKOUT
DURATION: 6 WEEKS OR AS NEEDED

Exercise	Exercise	Sets	Reps	Tempo/Hold	Weight	Rest	Notes
MUSCLE SPASM RELEASES – MYOFASCIAL RELEASE ON FOAM ROLLER							
#A1	Neck Release	1	2	10 secs			
#A4	Lower Back	2	1	20 secs			
#A5	Hips and ITB	2	1	15 secs			
#A6	Buttocks and Piriformis	2	1	20 secs			
#A7	Calf	1	1	15 secs			
#A8	Shins	1	1	10 secs			
#A9	Front Thigh	1	1	15 secs			
STRETCHES							
#B2	Neck – Side	1	1	10 secs			
#B3	Neck – Front	1	1	10 secs			
#B10	Lower Back	1	1	20 secs			
#B12	Russian Twist	1	10 total	313			
#B14	Hip and Inner Thigh	1	1	60 secs			Wall option
#B15	Calf	1	1	20 secs			
STABILITY ONLY							
#C4	Hip Extension – Outer Thigh	3	10	222		60 secs	Abduction with Swiss ball
#C5	Hip Extension – Inner Thigh	3	10	222		60 secs	Adduction with Swiss ball
#C7	4 Point Kneeling – Opposite Arm and Leg	3	10	424		60 secs	Only if comfortable on knees
#C9	Leg Lift – Swiss Ball	2	10	222		30 secs	

Notes:

No stretching is required after stability strength work.

This program is gentle enough for you to perform on most days of the week. You may wish to mix your week up with some swimming, or walking if you able to.

This program is only for 6 weeks; however you may wish to incorporate these stability exercises with your other programs. Check with your physical therapist and make sure you are doing these exercises correctly.

PROGRAM 37

SELF-MYOFASCIAL RELEASE BEFORE AND AFTER PREGNANCY

Exercise	Exercise	Times/Day	Sets	Reps	Hold	Rest	Followed by stretches in priority sequence
#A1	Neck Release	1	1	2	10 secs	nil	#B1, #B2, #B3, #B4 and #B5
#A2	Latissimus Dorsi	1	1	2	10 secs	nil	#B6, #B7 and #B8
#A3	Rhomboids	1	2	1	10 secs	nil	#B9
#A4	Lower Back	1-2	2	1	20 secs	nil	#B8, #B11, #B12 and #B10
#A5	Hips and ITB	1-2	2	1	15 secs	nil	#B13 and #B10
#A6	Buttocks and Piriformis	1-2	2	1	20 secs	nil	#B10
#A7	Calf	1	1	1	15 secs	nil	#B15
#A8	Shins	1	1	1	10 secs	nil	#B16
#A9	Front Thigh	1	1	1	15 secs	nil	#B13 and #B14

Notes:

This program lists all of the Self-Myofascial releases for before and after pregnancy. Choose as many as you feel would benefit you.

It is particularly effective to combine Self-Myofascial releases with stretching. I have identified the stretches that I would recommend after each release. Again, choose those that you feel would benefit you.

PROGRAM 38

STRETCHING EXERCISES FOR BEFORE AND AFTER PREGNANCY

Exercise	Exercise	Times/Day	Sets	Reps	Tempo/Hold	Rest	Notes
				Stretching			
#B1	Neck – Back	1	1	1	20 secs	nil	Contract-relax or just hold
#B2	Neck – Side	1	1	1	10 secs	nil	
#B3	Neck – Front	1	1	1	10 secs	nil	
#B4	Neck – Side	1	1	1	10 secs	nil	
#B5	Neck – Front	1	1	1	10 secs	nil	
#B6	Upper Back	1	1	1	20 secs	nil	
#B7	Upper Back	1	1	1	10 secs	nil	
#B8	Lower Back	1	1	1	10 secs	nil	Set may be repeated
#B9	Lower Back	1	2-3	1	10 sec	nil-30 secs	
#B10	Lower Back	1	1	1	20 secs	nil	Set may be repeated
#B11	McKenzie Press-up	1	1	10	323	nil	
#B12	Russian Twist	1	1	10	313	nil	
#B13	Hip and Thigh	1	2	1	10 secs	nil	Contract-relax or just hold
#B14	Hip and Inner Thigh	1	1	1	60 secs	nil	
#B15	Calf	1	1	1	20 secs	nil	
#B16	Shin	1	2	1	10 secs	nil	
#B17	Hamstring	1	2	1	20 secs	nil	

Notes:

This program lists all of the stretches for before and after pregnancy. Choose as many as you feel would benefit you.

PROGRAM 39

STABILITY EXERCISES FOR BEFORE AND AFTER PREGNANCY

Exercise	Exercise	Times/Day	Sets	Reps	Tempo/Hold	Rest	Notes
#C1	Hip Extension – Floor	1	1-3	10	323	nil-30secs	Rest if you are doing 3 sets
#C2	Hip Extension – Alternate Leg	1	2	10	5 secs	60 secs	Progression from #C1
#C3	Hip Extension – Swiss Ball	1	1-3	10	323	60 secs	
#C4	Hip Extension – Outer Thigh	1	2-3	10	222	0-60 secs	
#C5	Hip Extension – Inner Thigh	1	2-3	10	222	60 secs	
#C6	Basic 4 Point Kneeling	1	1-3	10	10 secs	60-120 secs	Beginner starts with 5 secs hold
#C7	4 Point Kneeling – Opposite Arm and Leg	1	2-3	10	424	60 secs	Progression from #C6
#C8	Superman	1	1-3	10	333	30-60 secs	Regression from #C7
#C9	Leg Lift – Swiss Ball	1	2	10	222	60 secs	
#C10	Prone Cobra – Swiss Ball	1	1-3	10	222	60 secs	
#C11	Lateral Ball Roll	1	1-2	8-12	slow	60 secs	Controlled move sideways

Notes:

This program lists all of the stability exercises for before and after pregnancy. Choose as many as you feel would benefit you.

PROGRAM 40

SELF-MYOFASCIAL RELEASE DURING PREGNANCY

Exercise	Exercise	Trimester	Sets	Reps	Intensity	Hold	Rest	Notes
#E1	Foot – Golf Ball	1 and 2	1	1	5/10	10 secs	nil	
#E2	Shins – Towel Grip	1, 2 and 3	2	10	5/10	N/A	nil	
#E3	ITB – Foam Roller	1 and 2	2	1	6/10	15 secs	10 secs	
#E4	Lats and Shoulders – Foam Roller	1 and 2	1	1	6/10	10 secs	10 secs	

Notes:

This program lists all of the Self-Myofascial releases during pregnancy. Choose as many as you feel would benefit you.

PROGRAM 41
STRETCHING DURING PREGNANCY

Exercise	Exercise	Trimesters	Sets	Reps	Hold	Rest	Notes
#F1	Calf – Wall	1, 2 and 3	1	1	20 secs	nil	See tips in #F1 for sciatic nerve pain
#F2	Achilles – Wall/Chair Version	1, 2 and 3	1	1	20 secs	nil	
#F3	Hamstrings	1, 2 and 3	1	1	20 secs	nil	
#F4	Inner Thigh	1, 2 and 3	1	1	20 secs	nil	
#F5	Piriformis – Hip	1, 2 and 3	2	1	20 secs	nil	
#F6	Quadriceps	1, 2 and 3	1	1	20 secs	nil	
#F7	Hip Flexor – Standing	1, 2 and 3	1	1	10 secs	nil	
#F8	Hip Flexor – Kneeling	1, 2 and 3	1	1	10-20 secs	nil	
#F9	Side Leg	1 and 2	1	1	10 secs	nil	
#F10	Lower Back and Waist	1 and 2	1	1	10-20 secs	nil	
#F11	Chest	1, 2 and 3	1	1	20 secs	nil	
#F12	Latissimus	1, 2 and 3	1	1	20 secs	nil	
#F13	Back	1 and 2	1	1	10 secs	nil	
#F14	Neck – Back	1, 2 and 3	1	1	20 secs	nil	
#F15	Neck – Side and Front	1, 2 and 3	1	1	20 secs	nil	
#F16	Neck – Back	1, 2 and 3	1	1	20 secs	nil	
#F17	Back and Breathing	1, 2 and 3	1	1	20 secs	nil	

Notes:

This program lists all of the stretches during pregnancy. Choose as many as you feel would benefit you.

PROGRAM 42
MOBILITY DURING PREGNANCY

Exercise	Exercise	Trimester	Sets	Reps	Tempo/ Hold	Rest	Notes
#G1	Lateral Pelvic Tilt	1, 2 and 3	2	20	slow	30 seconds	Move in a controlled manner
#G2	Anterior & Posterior Pelvic Tilt	1, 2 and 3	2	20	slow	30 seconds	
#G3	Lateral Pelvic Tilt – Kneeling	1, 2 and 3	2	20	slow	30 seconds	
#G4	Russian Twist	1 and 2	1-3	10	313	60 seconds	Move in a controlled manner
#G5	Muscle Energy Release	1 and 2	1-2	10	controlled	60 seconds	Breathing is key
#G6	Hip Extensions – Swiss Ball	1 and 2	1-3	8-12	222	60 seconds	
#G7	Hip Extension – Floor	1, 2 and 3	1-3	10	323	60 seconds	
#G8	Hip Extension – Towel	1, 2 and 3	1-3	10	323	60 seconds	
#G9	Buttock Squeeze -Tube	1 and 2	1-3	5-10	212	60 seconds	Controlled contraction

Notes:

This program lists all of the mobility exercises during pregnancy. Choose as many as you feel would benefit you.

GLOSSARY

Absolute contraindications

A woman should not participate in an exercise program during pregnancy if she has any of these conditions, unless otherwise prescribed by obstetrician.

Anterior

Front, or shifting forward.

Anterior vena cava

Large vein at the front of the hip/groin.

Blood pressure cuff

Blood pressure cuff, also known as a sphygmomanometer, is used as a tool to measure intra-abdominal pressure. For this purpose we want the manual version of those commonly used by doctors to measure your blood pressure. These are available from chemists, drugstores, medical equipment suppliers and even university bookshops. You may need to search a little to find a manual version, preferably with a needle, but this is best for our purposes. The one I have used is Heine Gamma 3.0 from Germany.

There is also another device called "Stabiliser" which you can purchase from PhysioRoom.com.

BOSU® – Dome

A piece of equipment that looks like a dome or a half ball that is used to provide an unstable platform for exercise. The top part is a heavy duty rubber that withstands load, while it sits on a plastic platform. BOSU® is used for balance, strength and stability exercises. You can perform exercises on the BOSU® using it dome side up or down.

Cardiac output

Volume of blood pumped by the heart.

Cervical extensors

Cervical extensors are muscles in the back of your neck. These can become tight and weak, hence the need for stretching and strengthening at the same time.

Cervical spine

The first 7 vertebrae of the spine (in the neck region).

Contract-relax method

Contract-relax stretch is a method where a muscle is placed under tension, without movement of the proximal (close) joint. Breathing through a Contract-relax stretch focuses you on your breathing, thereby increasing the value of the stretch. Holding the breath during a 5-count contract phase allows the muscle to go through tension, therefore when you breathe out, the release from tension allows the muscle greater stretch.

Core muscles (Transverse muscles, Pelvic floor muscles, Multifidus, Internal and External obliques)

The transverse muscles are "belt like" or "corset" muscles wrapped around the midsection of the body. They are the deepest of the major abdominal muscles with fibres running horizontally (transverse).

Multifidus is a deep spine muscle - a very thin muscle that runs from the base of the skull and all the way down to the tailbone. This muscle helps to support the spine vertebrae by vertebrae, but the only time it contracts is when the pelvic floor muscle is contracting. It also helps protect against degeneration of the joint structure.

Internal and External Obliques run diagonally across the body, and are the last muscles to activate during deep muscle contraction or intra-abdominal pressure.

Even though the diaphragm is not part of the "contraction" stage of the core muscles, it needs to be pointed out that when the diaphragm is working the pelvic floor muscles are relaxed. When the diaphragm is relaxed, the pelvic floor is contracting.

When I give instructions to connect the core muscles – I mean you should contract all the core muscles in at the same time.

DB

Dumbbells – hand weights used either in gym or home workouts.

Deep abdominal wall

The pressure or contraction in the deep abdominal wall is from the following muscles: transverse abdominals, pelvic floor, and multifidus.

Diaphragmatic breathing

Breathing diaphragmatically is using your diaphragm instead of your lungs. The diaphragm is located just under your ribcage. Focus on breathing in by lowering your diaphragm – your stomach will move outwards while your ribcage remains in the same position. Babies breathe predominantly from their diaphragm, as their lungs mature.

Drop sets

Performing an exercise using a certain amount of weight for an exercise until failure or exhaustion, reducing the weight and continuing to another failure and then reducing the weight again to another failure.

Extension

Straightening a joint or lengthening the body.

External rotation

Where the joint is rotated outwards e.g. feet pointing outward like a ballerina.

Feldenkrais method

Feldenkrais method offers gentle, relaxing and breathing movements' aimed to reduce pain or limitations in movement, to improve physical function, and to promote general wellbeing. Feldenkrais techniques are widely used in physical therapy and occupational therapy to treat muscle injuries, back pain and arthritis.

Flexion

Bending the body forward or closing a joint e.g. bowing down, bending the arm at the elbow, or bending the hip with the knee coming up.

Foam roller

A cylinder of hard foam roller, used for releasing tension in muscles. These are available from sports stores and physiotherapists.

Heart rate (HR)

Heart rate is measured as beats per minute (bpm).

Iliotibial Band (ITB)

The long fibrous tissue on the side of each thigh, glutes/hips, latissimus dorsi (long back muscles) and calves.

Incontinence

Weak pelvic floor muscles, leading to weak bladder control.

Internal rotation

Where the joint is rotated inwards e.g. knees will be closer together.

Kyphosis

Kyphosis in the spine refers to a rounded upper back.

Lumbar lordosis

Lumbar lordosis is an increase in the curvature of the lower back region. In pregnancy, the curve in the lower back increases due to the weight of the baby.

Lumbar spine

The lower portion of the spine consisting of 5 vertebrae. Lordosis in the spine refers to the increase in curvature.

Maximum Heart Rate (MHR)

Maximum heart rate is commonly calculated as follows: MHR = 220 - age.

Perceived Exertion Rate (RPE)

Perceived exertion rate is reported using the Borg scale and shows the intensity reported by a person by reference to a qualitative assessment of the difficulty of their exercise workload. It is commonly used to indicate the level of intensity of exercise that a person should perform.

Posterior

Back, or shifting backward.

Pronated

Rolling inwards e.g. collapsed arches or flat feet.

Protracted shoulder girdle

Protracted shoulder girdle means that you have a rounded upper back because all of the muscles around the shoulder blades are stretched. Exercises such as Prone Cobra should strengthen your shoulder blade muscles.

Psoas muscle

Psoas muscle is one of the hip flexor muscles. It originates from the lower spine and it attaches in the top of your thigh bone. It can be a problematic muscle, due to imbalanced workouts from the front and back of the body, causing a tight lower back.

Pubic Symphysis

Pubic Symphysis is the area just above a woman's clitoris. Pubic Symphysis issues during pregnancy include excessive movement in this area (either anterior or lateral) and associated pain, possibly because of an unstable pelvis.

Pyramiding

A strength training method where two exercises are chosen for each muscle group. Perform one or two warm up sets of 12 repetitions with light weight. Rest for 30 seconds after each warm up set. Follow with increasing weight for one set of 10 repetitions, one set of 8 repetitions, one set of 6 repetitions and immediately after the last set of 6, performing a set of 12 with light weight repetitions to reach a failure and fat burning effect.

Qi Qong method

Qi Qong is a traditional Chinese practice of breathing movements combined with specific exercises for therapeutic or healing purposes. Qi Qong (pronounced "Chi Gung") is from the family of Tai Chi, but is gentler with various breathing patterns to help the body with balance, strength, calm mind and visualisation of energising. Many Chinese believe it has healing properties.

Rectus abdominus

The rectus abdominus muscle is also commonly known as "abs" or "six pack". These are two parallel muscles running vertically, separated by a midline band of connective tissue.

Separation of the rectus abdominals occurs in more than 30% of women. Focus on strengthening the deep abdominal muscles instead as these have a huge role to play in the birth and post labour recovery.

Relative contraindications

A woman with any of these conditions should discuss with her obstetrician to modify the type of exercise program. Only proceed with exercise under supervision.

Relaxin

A hormone produced by the ovaries and the placenta. In preparation for childbirth, it relaxes the intrauterine ligaments in the pelvis, and softens and widens the cervix. During pregnancy, the hormone relaxin is present in 10 times its normal concentration – especially in the first trimester.

Round ligament pain

Round ligament pain is a sharp pain in their abdomen or hip area that may extend into the groin area. Round ligaments attach to the uterus around the area of the fallopian tubes.

Sciatica

Sciatica is nerve pain from irritation of the sciatic nerve. The pain is typically felt from the lower back (lumbar area) to behind the thigh and radiating down below the knee.

Super setting

This type of training is involves 2 exercises one after the other with no rest in between each set, involving same muscle group or opposing muscle groups.

Thoracic spine

The 12 vertebrae in the mid-section of the spine, below the cervical spine.

Toxemia

Toxemia of pregnancy is an abnormal condition characterised by hypertension (high blood pressure), edema (swelling) and protein in the urine.

Toxemia outside of pregnancy is blood poisoning caused by bacterial toxic substances in the blood.

Training effect

Training effect is when the body's metabolism is increased by exercise.

ACKNOWLEDGEMENTS

It is by God's grace that Pregnant, Fit and Fabulous has been birthed. Writing a book on a part-time basis while running two businesses had its challenges. I feel blessed to be surrounded by people with so much wisdom and gifting that have made my writing so much easier.

Alex and Stephanie, my beautiful girls, Mumma is in awe of you! Thank you for loving and believing in me, even when times were tough.

My Bacon family, mum Joan and late dad Sidney (who passed away suddenly before this printed edition was completed), for loving me like one of your own daughters... for always, always believing in me and encouraging me.

Thank you to my publishers Katherine Owen and DeeDee Heathman from GOKO Management and the Made for Success Team. You have been a dream to work with in bringing this book to publication.

Ruth Athanasio, my editor, thank you for your countless hours of editing and fine tuning everything. I will miss our Friday editing dates!

Stephanie Maddren, model, dancer and actor, thank you for being my amazing model. Your focus and professionalism in nailing every shot helped enormously.

Nikki Bullock, my gorgeous photographer, who took all my photos in the before and after pregnancy section.

George Fetting, from Headshot Factory, thank you for the amazing shoot with Stephanie Maddren. Your top notch experience and eye for detail is so valued.

David Hobbs, my assistant, words cannot describe my gratitude to you. I could not have done this without you. Thank you also to your lovely wife, Sue, who has been an amazing support and who has opened your home to me.

Mary Ferguson and Theresa Van der Velden, thanks for always being there for me and your great support.

Molly Knight, my herbalist and nutritionist, who inspired me to write this book.

To so many of my clients, too many to mention here, who inspire me daily! With your motivation and commitment to fitness - before, during and after pregnancy - may you always be Fit and Fabulous!

RESOURCES

Pregnant, Fit and Fabulous Website:
Visit *www.pregnantfitandfabulous.com* for updates, additional advice and further information.

Mary's Website:
Visit *www.marybacon.com* for other health and wellness information and speaking engagements.

Fitness Equipment:
Recommended equipment is available on *www.marybacon.com*

Pelvic Floor Physiotherapy and Pregnancy Training:
Penny Elliott - *www.physioposturefitness.com*

Continence, Pelvic Floor and Bladder Help:
Continence Foundation of Australia: *www.continence.org.au*

ABOUT THE AUTHOR

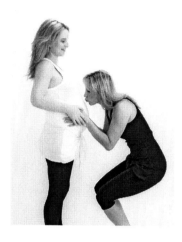

Based in Sydney, Mary is a qualified and registered Personal Fitness Trainer, Author of Pregnant Fit and Fabulous, Television & Radio Presenter and a corporate speaker. She works with some of Australia's leading health professionals, and recently publishing articles in Fitness First Magazine and leading newspapers.

She is a qualified and registered Personal Fitness trainer, Pregnancy-qualified specialist, Trigger Point therapist, and Sport Level 2 trainer.

An extraordinary fitness and nutrition expert with over 20 years experience, Mary Bacon's advice is sought after by Olympic medalists such as Jana Pittman, and the athletic elite as well as everyday people.

Mary's particular expertise is with pregnancy and fitness. Over many years, she has coached countless new mums to enjoy a happy and healthy pregnancy and their fit and fabulous pre and post-baby bodies. A genius at her craft, Mary has just revealed her wealth of proven health and fitness secrets for you in her sought-after new book, *Pregnant, Fit and Fabulous*.

Mary's passion is to help, inspire and influence people! Driven by results, Mary thrives on her clients exceeding their own expectations.

Humble at heart, she has a vision to impact and change the way women honour, think and love themselves.